STUDENT WORKBOOK TO ACCOMPANY

NURSING ASSISTANT

A Nursing Process Approach

11th Edition

W9-AFD-452

STUDENT WORKBOOK TO ACCOMPANY

NURSING ASSISTANT

A Nursing Process Approach

11th Edition

Barbara Acello, MS, RN
Independent Nurse Consultant and Educator

Barbara R. Hegner
(deceased)

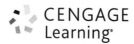

CENGAGE
Learning

Australia • Brazil • Japan • Korea • Mexico • Singapore • Spain • United Kingdom • United States

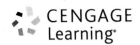
CENGAGE
Learning·

**Workbook to Accompany Nursing Assistant:
A Nursing Process Approach, 11th Edition,
Barbara Acello and Barbara R. Hegner**

SVP, GM Skills & Global Product
 Management: **Dawn Gerrain**

Associate Product Manager: **Laura Stewart**

Senior Director, Development: **Marah Bellegarde**

Product Development Manager: **Juliet Steiner**

Senior Content Developer: **Patricia Gaworecki**

Product Assistant: **Hannah Kinisky**

Vice President, Marketing Services:
 Jennifer Ann Baker

Marketing Manager: **Jonathan Sheehan**

Senior Director, Higher Education Content
 Production: **Wendy Troeger**

Production Director: **Andrew Crouth**

Senior Content Project Manager:
 Kenneth McGrath

Managing Art Director: **Jack Pendleton**

Cover image(s): © **Monkey Business Images/
 Shutterstock.com**

> For product information and technology assistance, contact us at
> **Cengage Learning Customer & Sales Support, 1-800-354-9706**
> For permission to use material from this text or product, submit all requests
> online at **www.cengage.com/permissions.**
> Further permissions questions can be e-mailed to
> **permissionrequest@cengage.com**

Library of Congress Control Number: 2014940408

ISBN: 978-1-133-13240-0

Cengage Learning
20 Channel Center Street
Boston, MA 02210
USA

Cengage Learning is a leading provider of customized learning solutions with office locations around the globe, including Singapore, the United Kingdom, Australia, Mexico, Brazil, and Japan. Locate your local office at: **www.cengage.com/global.**

Cengage Learning products are represented in Canada by Nelson Education, Ltd.

To learn more about Cengage Learning, visit **www.cengage.com**

Purchase any of our products at your local college store or at our preferred online store **www.cengagebrain.com**.

Notice to the Reader
Publisher does not warrant or guarantee any of the products described herein or perform any independent analysis in connection with any of the product information contained herein. Publisher does not assume, and expressly disclaims, any obligation to obtain and include information other than that provided to it by the manufacturer. The reader is expressly warned to consider and adopt all safety precautions that might be indicated by the activities described herein and to avoid all potential hazards. By following the instructions contained herein, the reader willingly assumes all risks in connection with such instructions. The publisher makes no representations or warranties of any kind, including but not limited to, the warranties of fitness for particular purpose or merchantability, nor are any such representations implied with respect to the material set forth herein, and the publisher takes no responsibility with respect to such material. The publisher shall not be liable for any special, consequential, or exemplary damages resulting, in whole or part, from the readers' use of, or reliance upon, this material.

Printed in the United States of America
Print Number: 01   Print Year: 2014

CONTENTS

The content of this workbook follows a basic organizational plan. Each lesson in the workbook includes:

- Behavioral objectives.
- A summary of the related unit in the *Nursing Assistant* text.
- Exercises to help you review, recall, and reinforce concepts that have been taught.
- Nursing Assistant Alerts, which are key points to remember about each unit.
- Opportunities to apply nursing assistant care to the nursing process and expand your horizons.

It has been shown that students who complete a special guide as they learn new materials perform better, have greater confidence, and are more secure in the basic concepts than those who do not. You may wish to complete the workbook activities in preparation for your class, or after class, while the information is fresh in your mind. In either case, the workbook and classwork will reinforce each other.

You can make the best use of the workbook if you:

- Read and study the related chapter in the text.
- Observe and listen carefully to your instructor's explanations and demonstrations.
- Read over the behavioral objectives before you start the workbook and then check to be sure you have met them after you complete the lesson exercises.
- Use the summary to review the chapter content.
- Complete the activities in the workbook. Circle any questions you are unable to finish to discuss with your instructor at the next class meeting.

You have chosen a special goal for yourself: You have decided to become a knowledgeable, skilled nursing assistant. Keep this goal in mind, but realize that to reach it, you need to take many small steps. Each step you master takes you closer to your ultimate goal. Best wishes as you embark on your journey!

Barbara Acello

THE LEARNING PROCESS

Students may feel anxious about learning. However, learning really can be very rewarding if you have an open mind, a desire to succeed, and a willingness to follow some simple steps.

You already have won half the battle, because you have entered an educational program. This shows your desire to accomplish a real-life goal: to become a nursing assistant.

Steps to Learning

There are three basic steps to learning:

- Active listening
- Effective studying
- Careful practicing

Active Listening

Listening actively is not easy, natural, or passive. It is, however, a skill that can be learned and must be practiced.

Good listeners are not born, they are made. Studies show that the average listening efficiency in this culture is only about 25 percent. That means that although you may hear (a passive action) all that is said, you actually listen to and process only about one-quarter of the material. Effective listening requires a conscious effort by the listener. The most neglected communication skill is listening.

An important part of your work as a nursing assistant involves active listening to patients and co-workers. Begin to listen actively to your instructor or supervisor. Hearing but not processing information puts you and your patient in jeopardy.

Active listening is listening with personal involvement. There are three actions in active listening:

- Hearing what is said (passive action)
- Processing the information (active action)
- Using the information (active action)

Hearing What Is Said

People speak at an average rate of 125 words per minute. Pay close attention to the speaker to hear what is said. This is not difficult if you focus and do not let other thoughts and sounds interfere with your thinking. If you sit up straight and lean forward in the classroom or stand erect in the clinical area, your whole body is more receptive. Position yourself where you can adequately see or hear and keep your attention focused on the speaker. Make eye contact if possible and remain alert.

Many distractions can break your concentration unless you actively prevent them from doing so. For example, distractions may be:

- Interruptions, such as other activities in the classroom or in the patient's unit that catch your attention or create noise.
- Daydreaming and thinking about personal activities or problems.

- Physical fatigue. Adequate sleep and rest are powerful aids to the ability to concentrate.

- Lack of interest, because you cannot immediately see the importance of the information.

To be an effective listener, you must actively work at eliminating these distractions. You must put energy into staying focused.

Processing the Information

Remember that hearing the words is not enough. You must actively process (make sense of) the words in your brain by putting meaning to them, and that takes effort. Other things can also help the process, including:

- Interacting with the speaker using eye contact, smiles, and nods.

- Asking meaningful questions; contribute your own comments if it is a discussion.

- Taking notes.

These actions allow your memory to establish relationships with previously learned knowledge and to make new connections.

Taking notes gives you another way to imprint what you are processing. You are not only hearing the sounds of the words, but also seeing the important words on paper. Note-taking helps you recall points that you may have forgotten.

Note-taking is a skill that can be learned. If used, it will greatly improve your learning process. You may need to take notes in class, during demonstrations, and when your supervisor or instructor gives you a clinical assignment. Here are some hints to make developing this skill easier:

- Come prepared with a pencil and paper.

- Don't try to write down every word.

- Write down only the important points or key words.

- Learn to take notes in an outline form.

- Listen with particular care to the beginning sentence. It usually reveals the primary purpose.

- Pay special attention to the final statement. It is often a summary.

Outlines include the important points summarized in a meaningful way. Be sure to leave room so that you can add material.

There are different ways of outlining. One way is to use letters and numbers to designate important points. Another is to draw a pattern of lines to show relationships. Use either way or one of your own design, but be consistent. Practice helps you master the skill of outlining.

As you make notes of material that is not clear, add a star or some other mark next to the material. When the speaker asks for questions, you can quickly find yours.

If the speaker stresses a point, underline the information to call attention to important points to study.

After class, you can reorganize your notes and compare them with your text.

GENERAL TIPS

Here are some general tips to help you study better.

- Feel certain that each lesson you master is important to add to your knowledge and skills. The workbook, text, and instructor materials have been carefully coordinated to meet the objectives. Review the objectives before you begin to study. They are like a road map that will take you to your goal.

- Remember that you are the learner, so you can take credit for your success. The instructor is an important guide and the workbook, text, and clinical experiences are tools, but you are the learner and whether you use the tools wisely is up to you in the end.

- Take an honest look at yourself and your study habits. Take positive steps to avoid habits that could limit your success. For example, do you let family responsibilities or social opportunities interfere with study times? If so, sit down with your family and plan a schedule for study that they will support and to which you will adhere. Find a special place to study that is free from distraction. If the telephone interferes, turn it off.

The Study Plan

Plan a schedule for study. Actually sit down and write out a weekly schedule hour by hour so that you know exactly how your time is being spent. Then plan specific study time, but be realistic. Study must be balanced with the other activities of your life. Learn to budget your time so that you have time to study. Block in extra time when tests are scheduled. Don't forget to block in time for fun as well! Look back over the week to see how well you have managed your schedule. If you have had difficulty, try to adjust the schedule to better meet your needs. If you have been successful, pat yourself on the back. You have done very well.

Make your study area special. It need not be elaborate, but make sure there is ample light. You should have a desk to work on and a supply of paper and pencils. Sharpen your pencils at the end of each study period and leave papers readily at hand. You may think this sounds strange, but often time is wasted at the beginning of a study session finding paper and sharpening pencils. If these things are ready when you first sit down, you can get started without distractions or delay. Keep your medical dictionary and other references in your work area. When you get home, put your text and workbook there also. In other words, your work area should be designed for study. When you treat it this way, you will find that as soon as you sit down there, you will be psychologically prepared to study.

Class Study

Now that you have your study area and work schedule organized, you need to think about how you can get the most out of your class experience.

- Come prepared. Read the behavioral objectives and the lesson before class. This introduces you to the focus of the lesson and the vocabulary.

- Listen actively as the instructor explains the lesson. Pay close attention. Refocus immediately if your thoughts start to wander.

- Take notes on the special points to use for study at home.

- Participate in class discussions. Remember that discussion subjects are chosen because they relate to the lesson. You can learn much from hearing the comments of others and by contributing your own. Pay attention to slides, films, and overhead transparencies, because these offer a visual approach to the subject matter. You might even take notes on important points during a film or jot down questions you would like the instructor to answer.

- Ask intelligent and pertinent questions. Make sure your questions are simple and centered on the topic. Focus on one point at a time and write down the answers for later review.

- Use any models and charts that are available. Study them and see how they apply to the lesson.

- Carefully observe the demonstrations your instructor gives. Note in your book any change that may have been made in the procedure steps to conform with the policy of your facility.

- Perform return demonstrations carefully in the classroom. Remember, you are learning skills that will be used with real patients in the clinical situation.

After Class

When class is over and you have had a break, you are ready to settle down and study. You can gain the most from the experience by:

- Studying in your prepared study area. Everything will be ready and waiting for you if you followed the first part of this plan.

- Read over the lesson, beginning with the behavioral objectives.

- Read with a highlighter or pencil in hand so you can underline or highlight important material.

- Answer the questions at the end of the unit. Check any you found difficult by reviewing that section of the text.

- Complete the related workbook unit.

- Review the behavioral objectives at the beginning of the unit. Ask yourself if you have met them. If not, go back and review. Prepare the next day's lesson by reading over the next day's unit.

- Use the medical dictionary for words you may learn that are not in the text glossary. The dictionary provides pronunciations.

Study Groups

Studying with someone else who is trying to learn the same material can be very helpful and supportive, but there are some pitfalls you must avoid. If studying with someone else is to be effective and productive:

- Limit the number of people studying to a maximum of three; one other person is best.

- Keep focused on the subject. Don't begin to talk about classmates or the day's social events.

- Come prepared for the study session. Have your work completed. Use the study session to reinforce your learning and explore deeper understanding of the material.

- Ask each other questions about the materials.

- Make a list of ideas to ask your instructor.

- Limit the study session to a specific length. Follow the plan and you will succeed!

STUDY SKILLS

OBJECTIVES

After completing this unit, you will be able to:

- Spell and define terms.
- Describe the effect of study skills on successful learning.
- Write the steps involved in active listening.
- List interferences to effective listening.
- Use two techniques of note-taking.
- Name ways to improve study habits.
- Effectively use the textbook.

UNIT SUMMARY

Developing effective study habits can be important to a lifetime of learning. A few simple steps can make the process easier.

- Become familiar with your text. It will save time in locating information.
- Practice the steps to learning by being an active listener.
- Take notes for reference and study.
- Plan study times and practice in ways that promote learning.

ACTIVITIES

Vocabulary Exercise

Define the words in the spaces provided.

1. active listening

2. end-of-unit materials

3. processing

4. behavioral objectives

_____

5. glossary

_____

Completion

Complete the statements in the spaces provided.

1. Behavioral objectives help to direct your _____.

2. There are three basic steps to learning: _____, _____, and _____.

3. Daydreaming can _____ with your ability to listen actively.

4. Planning a schedule of classes and other responsibilities will help you use study time more
   _____.

5. Use the _____ to learn the meaning of new terms and words.

6. Follow the maze. Which path will you travel?

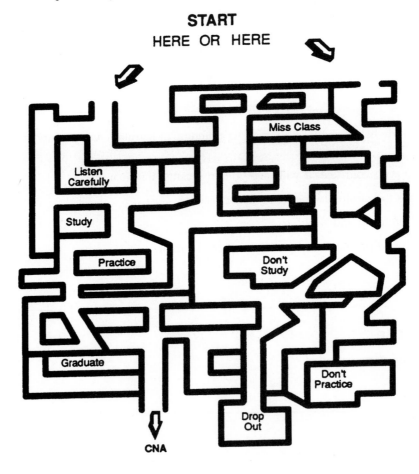

7. Name techniques of note-taking.

   a. _____

   b. _____

8. Read the following case history. Then use one of the two note-taking techniques to outline the material.

Victoria Bohn was 8½ months pregnant when she first appeared at our family planning clinic. The mother of three lively little girls, ages 13 months, 2 years, and 3 years, she looked tired as her children pulled at her skirts and fussed.

When her turn came to be examined, the nursing assistant found that her blood pressure was 148/100, pulse 92, respiration 24, temperature 103°F. Her hands and fingers were swollen, and she complained of pain in her abdomen high on the right side. She had gained 38 pounds since becoming pregnant. Concerned, the nursing assistant informed the nurse.

After examining Ms. Bohn and listening to her baby's heartbeat, Mrs. Edelson, the registered nurse supervising the clinic, told Ms. Bohn that she wanted her to be seen by the physician. When the physician made his examination, he immediately recommended that Ms. Bohn be admitted to the acute care hospital.

During her hospitalization, it was found that the patient had a severe infection in her abdomen, which was successfully treated with antibiotics. While in the hospital, her blood pressure and fluid levels were brought within normal limits.

Ms. Bohn remained in the hospital until delivery of a beautiful 8-pound girl. A grandmother, who had been helping take care of the family, agreed to remain in the home for a period of time until Ms. Bohn was once again able to manage her family herself.

Student Activities

Introduction to Nursing Assisting

Community Health Care

OBJECTIVES

After completing this unit, you will be able to:

- Spell and define terms.
- List the five basic functions of health care facilities.
- Describe four changes that have taken place in health care in the past few decades.
- State the functions of hospitals, long-term care facilities, home health care, hospice, and other types of health care facilities.
- Name the departments within a hospital and describe their functions.
- List at least five ways by which health care costs are paid.
- State the purpose of health care facility surveys.
- Describe patient-focused care.
- Explain why transitional care is important.

UNIT SUMMARY

- Health care facilities provide health care to members of the community.
- Specific care is provided in different types of facilities.
- Patient-focused care emphasizes and concentrates on the unique needs of each person.
- Nursing assistants play an important role in this caregiving.

- Many changes have occurred within the past few years, brought about by an aging population, new technologies, and the need to contain costs.
- Persons with different types of experience and training work as a team to meet each person's health needs.
- Health care facilities must comply with health and safety laws and regulations, and undertake activities to ensure quality.

ACTIVITIES

Vocabulary Exercise

Define the words in the spaces provided.

1. facility

   _____

2. hospice

   _____

3. patient

   _____

4. transitional care

   _____

5. community

   _____

Completion

Complete the statements in the spaces provided.

1. List five basic functions of all health care facilities.

   a. _____

   b. _____

   c. _____

   d. _____

   e. _____

2. Patient-focused care means

   _____

   _____.

3. The cost of health care has increased because of demand for services as a result of

   _____

   _____.

4. The person receiving care in an acute care hospital is called a

   _____

   _____.

5. List three examples of health care facilities.

   a. _____

   b. _____

   c. _____

6. Three names applied to the person receiving care are:

   a. _____

   b. _____

   c. _____

7. Explain what activities take place in each of the following departments.

   a. pharmacy

   _____

   b. medical

   _____

   c. radiology

   _____

   d. pediatric

   _____

   e. physical therapy

   _____

8. Explain the activities of each of the following departments.

   a. dietary

   _____

   b. housekeeping

   _____

   c. maintenance

   _____

   d. business

   _____

9. List four ways volunteers help patients.

   a. _____

   b. _____

   c. _____

   d. _____

10. The majority of health care is paid for with

   _____

11. The purpose of diagnosis related groups is to

   _____

12. A health care facility survey is done to

   _____

13. The Occupational Safety and Health Administration is a governmental agency that

   _____

Word Search

1. Find the following words in the puzzle. Put a circle around each word and define each in the spaces provided.

```
R W Z I K G B Q C W F P Y C
P E L R J C A U D K O E H I
R P H U E T Y Q I S V K O T
E A C A Q Z E R T R B M S A
N T O A B A R P U J L N P T
A I I V H I A S Z I H U I I
T E G U U R L R K Y R B C O
A N Y R T V F I T T N B E N
L T M U K G V A T Q V Q L H
B X M S A J M E R A H I A K
Q B O D B K C J Y T T G G E
Z P R Q C I N O R H C I W X
V L R X Y T I L I C A F O E
P A T H O L O G Y J B J V N
```

a. hospice

_____

b. postpartum

_____

c. prenatal

_____

d. pathology

_____

e. facility

_____

f. survey

_____

g. rehabilitation

_____

h. citation

_____

i. chronic

_____

j. patient

_____

DEVELOPING GREATER INSIGHT

1. Visit a local community health agency such as a city or county health department and learn about its services. Report back to the class.

2. Accompany a volunteer in a hospital. Learn about the volunteer's work and see how many departments you can identify.

3. Make a list of the health care facilities within your immediate vicinity and identify the type of care provided in each.

4. Invite a nursing assistant who is currently employed by a health care facility to visit the class and discuss the care provided by nursing assistants in that facility. An alternate activity is to prepare a list of questions about the role and responsibilities of the nursing assistant. Interview a nursing assistant, then discuss the responses with your class.

On the Job: Being a Nursing Assistant

OBJECTIVES

After completing this unit, you will be able to:

- Spell and define terms.
- Identify the members of the interdisciplinary health care team and the nursing team.
- List the job responsibilities of the nursing assistant, explain how the Nurse Practice Act affects nursing assistant practice, and discuss the importance of working within the established scope of nursing assistant practice.
- List the federal requirements for nursing assistants working in long-term care facilities.
- State the purpose of evidence-based practice.
- Identify common nursing care delivery systems and briefly describe each.
- Describe your facility's lines of authority and discuss the five rights of delegation.
- Explain why good time management is a key to nursing assistant success and describe methods of organizing assignments to make the best use of your time.
- State the purpose of shift report and handoff communication.
- Describe the importance of good human relations and list ways of building good relationships with patients, families, and staff.
- Discuss professionalism and explain why projecting a professional image is important.
- List the rules of personal hygiene and appropriate dress.
- Describe ways to prevent physical illness and relieve stress, and the importance of a healthy mental attitude.

UNIT SUMMARY

Nursing assistants:

- Have specific responsibilities that vary within different agencies, but must always function within the scope of nursing assistant practice.

- Must follow established procedures and policies.

- Represent themselves and the agency or facility; therefore, good grooming is essential.

- Are responsible for their own actions.

- Must develop good interpersonal relationships with patients, visitors, and co-workers.

- Will find that personal adjustments are made easier by understanding and obeying facility policies and procedures.

- Must always treat patients, co-workers, and visitors with dignity.

- Must take a written or oral and clinical (skills) test to become certified.

- May be cross-trained to increase their skills.

NURSING ASSISTANT ALERT

Action	**Benefit**
Maintain good grooming.	Enhances appearance and health. Inspires patient confidence.
Make sure uniform is complete.	Identifies your role and responsibilities.
Practice stress reduction.	Keeps you mentally and emotionally stable.

ACTIVITIES

Vocabulary Exercise

Define the words in the spaces provided.

1. attitude

_____

2. burnout

_____

3. nursing team

_____

4. scope of practice

_____

5. nursing assistant

_____

6. partners in practice

_____

Completion

Complete the statements in the spaces provided.

1. Write four terms used to describe the nursing assistant.

    a. _____

    b. _____

    c. _____

    d. _____

2. List three members of the nursing team.

    a. _____

    b. _____

    c. _____

3. Explain what is meant by the "line of authority."

    _____

    _____

4. What should you do if you have any doubts about your assignment?

    _____

5. State the three primary ways in which nursing care is organized and give a brief explanation of each.

    a. primary nursing _____

    _____

    b. case management _____

    _____

    c. team nursing _____

    _____

6. List three goals of patient-focused care.

    a. _____

    b. _____

    c. _____

7. Name three characteristics of a successful nursing assistant.

    a. _____

    b. _____

    c. _____

8. List three activities you could carry out to ensure good personal hygiene.

    a. _____

    b. _____

    c. _____

9. Explain why wearing jewelry is unwise when you are on duty.

    _____

    _____

10. What jewelry is part of your uniform?

    _____

11. The main concern of every nursing assistant should be the well-being and

    _____.

12. List four reasons why a patient might be irritable, complaining, or uncooperative.

    a. _____

    b. _____

    c. _____

    d. _____

13. List three dimensions in which patients have needs.

    a. _____

    b. _____

    c. _____

14. List five ways you can ensure good working relationships.

    a. _____

    b. _____

    c. _____

    d. _____

    e. _____

15. Check the positive and negative grooming traits of a nursing assistant.

Trait	Positive	Negative
a. long hair		
b. clean shoelaces		
c. cigarette odor		
d. bright nail polish		
e. unpolished shoes		
f. dangling earrings		
g. light lipstick		
h. long fingernails		
i. use of antiperspirant/deodorant		

16. Explain why stress is an issue for all nursing assistants and how you can reduce its effects.

_____

_____

_____

17. Define:

   a. Palliative care

   _____

   b. Cross-training

   _____

18. Complete the chart to show the proper lines of communication.

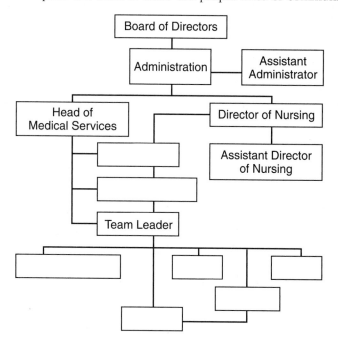

Matching

Match the specialist and the type of care provided.

Type of Care

1. _____ Care of the aging person
2. _____ Treats and diagnoses disorders of the eye
3. _____ Treats disorders of the skin
4. _____ Treats disorders of the digestive system
5. _____ Treats disorders of the heart and blood vessels
6. _____ Treats and diagnoses disorders of the nervous system
7. _____ Treats disorders of the blood
8. _____ Cares for women during pregnancy
9. _____ Diagnoses and treats with X-rays
10. _____ Treats disorders of the mind

Specialist

a. Cardiologist
b. Gastroenterologist
c. Neurologist
d. Radiologist
e. Obstetrician
f. Hematologist
g. Psychiatrist
h. Ophthalmologist
i. Gerontologist
j. Dermatologist

DEVELOPING GREATER INSIGHT

1. With other students, role-play a properly dressed and improperly dressed nursing assistant. State your first impressions about each assistant based on how he or she is dressed. Discuss how this influences your feelings about the person. Divide the class into teams and assign points for each positive or negative finding.

2. With the class, discuss ways you have personally found to relieve stress. Discuss why alcohol and other drugs are a poor solution to stress.

3. Discuss burnout, what it feels like, and how people behave when they experience it. Try to learn what effect it might have on the burned-out individual, co-workers, and patients.

Consumer Rights and Responsibilities in Health Care

OBJECTIVES

After completing this unit, you will be able to:

- Spell and define terms.
- Explain the purpose of health care consumer rights.
- Describe six items that are common to the Patient Care Partnership booklet, the Resident's Rights, and the Client's Rights in Home Care documents.
- List three specific rights from each of the three documents.
- State the purpose of the Affordable Care Act and review the new Patient's Bill of Rights under that law.
- Describe eight responsibilities of health care consumers.

UNIT SUMMARY

Consumer rights protect patients and ensure optimum care. They are spelled out in special documents such as:

- Patient Care Partnership Clients' Rights in Home Care
- Residents' Rights

Consumer rights are protected and optimal care is better ensured when consumers participate in the process by:

- Sharing health histories openly

- Participating in their own care to the extent possible
- Accepting financial responsibility
- Being sure they understand care directions
- Living a healthful lifestyle

NURSING ASSISTANT ALERT

Action	Benefit
Understand and be guided by consumer rights	Protects patients. Ensures optimal care.

ACTIVITIES

Vocabulary Exercise

Using the definitions, unscramble the words that identify documents designed to protect consumers of health care. Write the words in the blanks.

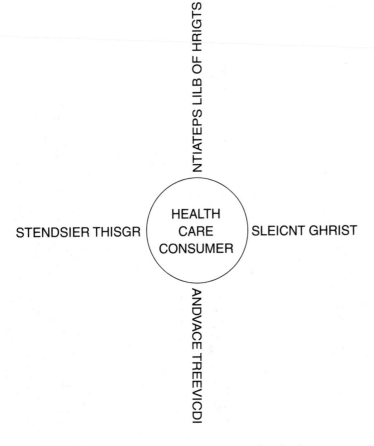

NTIATEPS LILB OF HRIGTS

STENDSIER THISGR

HEALTH CARE CONSUMER

SLEICNT GHRIST

ANDVACE TREEVICDI

1. Given to patients upon admission to a hospital

   _____

2. Relates to people receiving care at home

   _____

3. Given to people before admission to a long-term care facility

   _____

4. Gives instructions about consumers' wishes regarding care when they are unable to make their wishes known

   _____

Ethical and Legal Issues Affecting the Nursing Assistant

OBJECTIVES

After completing this unit, you will be able to:

- Spell and define terms.
- Discuss ethical and legal situations in health care.
- Describe the legal and ethical responsibilities of the nursing assistant.
- Describe how to protect patients' right to privacy.
- Define abuse and neglect, and give examples of each.
- Define sexual harassment and give examples of activities that may be perceived as being sexually harassing.
- Identify professional boundaries in relationships with patients and families.
- Explain why working in a virtual world affects patient boundaries and give examples of boundary violations using the Internet and wireless media.
- State the purpose of the HIPAA laws.
- Explain why most facilities prohibit employees from posting work-related information on social networking sites.

UNIT SUMMARY

All persons giving health care voluntarily adhere to a set of ethical standards. They agree to:

- Protect life
- Promote health
- Keep personal information confidential

- Respect personal death beliefs
- Give care based on need, not gratuities (tips)
- Provide safety

17

Nursing assistants have legal responsibilities. Legal situations the health care provider wants to avoid include:

- Negligence
- Assault and battery
- Theft
- Invasion of privacy
- Abuse
- Malpractice
- Neglect

NURSING ASSISTANT ALERT

Action	Benefit
Maintain ethical standards.	Protects patients' rights and privacy.
Obey laws.	Protects you against legal actions and keeps patient safe.
Carry out orders or report inability to do so to supervisor.	Ensures proper and safe nursing care.
Protect patients' physical and personal privacy.	Promotes patients' sense of security. Makes patients feel secure and protected.
Applies the Platinum Rule.	Ensures that patients have a voice in their care.
Stays within the zone of helpfulness.	Helps maintain healthy relationships with patients.
Uses good judgment in working in a virtual world.	Maintains confidentiality of patients and the employer.
Applies HIPAA rules.	Restricts use and avoids disclosure of patient information.

ACTIVITIES

Vocabulary Exercise

Define the words in the spaces provided.

1. confidential

   _____

2. assault

   _____

3. negligence

   _____

4. verbal abuse

   _____

5. slander

   _____

6. malpractice

_____

7. neglect

_____

Completion

Complete the statements in the spaces provided.

1. Ethical standards are a _____ code rather than a legal code.

2. List five ways to ensure that the patient receives the proper treatment.

   a. _____

   b. _____

   c. _____

   d. _____

   e. _____

3. The patient offers you a tip for going to the lobby to get him a newspaper from the machine. Describe and explain your response.

   _____

   _____

4. You have not stolen something belonging to a patient yourself, but you observed someone else do so and failed to report it. Of what crime are you guilty?

   _____

5. A visitor asks you if her father really has cancer. How should you respond?

   _____

6. Restraining a patient without proper permission is _____

   _____

7. Abuse is any act that is not _____ and causes harm to the patient.

8. A door that is shut against a patient's will when the patient is confined to bed is a form of

   _____

9. Define the Golden Rule.

   _____

   _____

10. Define the Platinum Rule.

   _____

   _____

11. You are in the _____ when you get too close to a boundary.

```
            |                    |
            |    Zone of         |   _____
            |                    |
  ◄─────────┼────────────────────┼──────────►
            |                    |
   _____|    Helpfulness      |
            |                    |
```

12. Label the professional behavior continuum in the figure.

True/False

Mark the following true or false by circling T or F.

1. T F It is the responsibility of a nursing assistant to determine whether a patient has been abused.
2. T F A nursing assistant who reports seeing bruises or injuries on a patient is acting properly.
3. T F Self-abuse may occur when a disabled person is unable to adequately carry out ADLs and will not accept help.
4. T F Signs of poor personal hygiene and a change of personality may indicate abuse.
5. T F Most abuse originates in feelings of frustration and fatigue.
6. T F An employee assistance program has resources to help reduce stress.
7. T F Separation of a patient may be permitted if it is part of a therapeutic plan to reduce agitation.
8. T F A nursing assistant may independently decide to isolate a patient.
9. T F In some states, a person who does not report abuse is held as guilty as the abusing person.
10. T F You may write about patients on your blog as long as you alter their names.
11. T F Employee behavior reflects upon the employer, even if the employee is not on duty.
12. T F You leave footprints that can be traced whenever you use the Internet.
13. T F Loretta forgot to feed Mr. Locklear his lunch. This is a form of neglect.

Complete the Chart

Place an X in the appropriate space to show which type of abuse has taken place.

Action	Verbal Abuse	Sexual Abuse	Psychological Abuse	Physical Abuse
1. Touching a patient in a sexual way	—	—	—	—
2. Using obscene gestures	—	—	—	—
3. Raising your voice in anger	—	—	—	—
4. Teasing a patient	—	—	—	—
5. Handling a patient roughly	—	—	—	—
6. Making threats	—	—	—	—
7. Making fun of the patient	—	—	—	—

(continues)

Action	Verbal Abuse	Sexual Abuse	Psychological Abuse	Physical Abuse
8. Ridiculing a patient's behavior	—	—	—	—
9. Suggesting that the patient engage in sexual acts with you	—	—	—	—
10. Hitting a patient	—	—	—	—
11. Leaving the patient in bed when she asks repeatedly to get up	—	—	—	—
12. Holding an alert patient down when the nurse performs a dressing change against her will	—	—	—	—
13. Seating an alert patient at a table with three confused patients, rather than seating her in an empty spot at a table with three alert patients	—	—	—	—
14. Wiping a female patient internally with a washcloth while doing routine perineal care	—	—	—	—
15. Turning a sleeping patient with no warning	—	—	—	—
16. Saying, "If you don't stop using the call signal so much, I am not going to bring your lunch tray."	—	—	—	—
17. Unplugging the patient's call signal because she is making too many minor requests	—	—	—	—
18. Deliberately arousing a confused male patient when applying a condom catheter	—	—	—	—

Scientific Principles

Medical Terminology and Body Organization

OBJECTIVES

After completing this unit, you will be able to:

- Spell and define terms.
- Recognize the meanings of common prefixes, suffixes, and root words.
- Build medical terms from word parts.
- Write the abbreviations commonly used in health care facilities.
- Describe the organization of the body, from simple to complex.
- Name four types of tissues and their characteristics.
- Name and locate major organs as parts of body systems, using proper anatomic terms.

UNIT SUMMARY

Medical terminology is developed by arranging and combining word parts. It is a language used by personnel in health care facilities. The words are formed of:

- Word roots
- Prefixes at the beginning of words
- Suffixes at the end of words
- Combining forms referring to body parts and medical actions

- Abbreviations (usually letters)

The human body is organized into:

- Various kinds of cells
- Four basic tissue types
- Many organs
- 10 systems

Each contributes in a special way to the total structure and physiology of the body. A careful study of the healthy body and its organization provides a foundation for learning about your own body and the bodies of your patients. Learning medical terminology will improve your understanding, help you communicate more effectively in the health care setting, and improve your accuracy in reporting and documenting your observations.

NURSING ASSISTANT ALERT

Action	Benefit
Analyze medical and scientific terms.	Improves comprehension. Increases vocabulary. Improves communication skills.
Practice using combining forms.	Increases verbal and written skills.
Study the anatomy and physiology of the body.	Improved understanding of normal body structure and functions.
Learn proper names for body parts.	Allows more accurate communication of observations.

ACTIVITIES

Vocabulary Exercise

Define the words in the spaces provided.

1. prefix

   _____

2. suffix

   _____

3. abbreviation

   _____

4. combining form

   _____

5. word root

   _____

Completion

Complete the statements in the spaces provided.

1. Name the book, other than your text, that would be most helpful in studying medical terms.

   _____

2. Underline the <u>root</u> in each of the following words and give a definition of the word.

   Example: <u>abdomin</u>al   pertaining to the abdomen

   a. adenoma _____

   b. colectomy _____

   c. craniotomy _____

   d. dentist _____

   e. hysterectomy _____

   f. myalgia _____

   g. nephrolithiasis _____

   h. pneumonectomy _____

   i. thoracotomy _____

   j. urinometer _____

3. Underline the <u>prefix</u> in each of the following words and give a definition of the prefix.

   Example: <u>neo</u>plasm   new

   a. asepsis _____

   b. bradycardia _____

   c. dysuria _____

   d. hypertension _____

   e. hypotension _____

   f. pandemic _____

   g. polyuria _____

   h. gerontology _____

   i. premenstrual _____

   j. tachycardia _____

4. Underline the <u>suffix</u> in each of the following words and give a definition of the suffix.

   Example: acro<u>megaly</u>   great

   a. appendectomy _____

   b. hepatitis _____

   c. electrocardiogram _____

   d. anemia _____

   e. tracheotomy _____

   f. hematology _____

   g. hemiplegia _____

   h. apnea _____

   i. otoscope _____

   j. proctoscopy _____

5. Listed below are five words not in your text. Define each and then check your accuracy with a medical dictionary.

   a. adenitis

   _____

   b. cardiopathy

   _____

   c. leukopenia

   _____

   d. arthroscope

   _____

   e. cytomegaly

   _____

6. Substitute one word for the underlined words in each of the following statements.

   Example: The patient experienced <u>pus in the urine</u>.   pyuria

   a. There was <u>sugar in the urine</u>. _____

   b. The patient made an appointment with a <u>physician who specializes in female diseases</u>.

   _____

   c. The nurse performed a <u>puncture in a vein</u> and drew blood.

   _____

   d. The patient has an <u>incision made into the trachea</u> to ease breathing.

   _____

   e. The patient had a <u>tumor composed mainly of fibrous tissue</u> removed from her uterus.

   _____

   f. The patient was receiving chemotherapy for cancer, which caused <u>depression of all her cell levels</u>.

   _____

   g. The nursing assistant listened with the stethoscope to the patient's heart. She found <u>the heart rate was slow</u>.

   _____

   h. The medication did not seem to help the patient's <u>high blood pressure</u>.

   _____

   i. The postoperative diagnosis was <u>removal of a lung</u>. _____

   j. The patient complained of pain <u>under the stomach</u>. _____

7. Explain the following diagnoses.

   a. thrombosis

   _____

   b. pyogenic infection

   _____

  c. pneumonitis

_____

  d. cystitis

_____

  e. mastitis

_____

8. Write the name of the body part indicated by the abbreviation.

  a. abd _____

  b. bld _____

  c. G.I. _____

  d. AX _____

  e. GU _____

  f. vag _____

  g. sh _____

Matching

Match the letters on the left with the medical diagnosis on the right.

1. _____ AIDS
2. _____ CHF
3. _____ CVA
4. _____ Fx
5. _____ TIA
6. _____ MI
7. _____ HCV
8. _____ KS
9. _____ STD
10. _____ MS

a. fracture

b. transient ischemic attack

c. hepatitis C virus

d. multiple sclerosis

e. acquired immune deficiency syndrome

f. nonspecific urethritis

g. sexually transmitted disease

h. cerebrovascular accident

i. Kaposi's sarcoma

j. myocardial infarction

k. congestive heart failure

Abbreviations

The following is a list of abbreviations you will see relating to orders and patient care. Write your understanding of each abbreviation.

1. a. amb. ad lib. _____

  b. urine to lab ASAP _____

  c. BR only _____

    d. ✔ drsg freq _____

    e. OOB daily _____

    f. position HOB 45° _____

    g. d/c cl liq diet _____

    h. SSE prn _____

    i. CBC in AM _____

    j. NPO preop _____

2. Write the names of the following hospital departments.

    a. CS _____

    b. EENT _____

    c. PT _____

    d. ICCU _____

    e. ED _____

    f. PAR _____

    g. Peds _____

    h. DR _____

    i. OR _____

    j. Lab _____

3. Write the appropriate abbreviation for the time indicated.

    a. before meals _____

    b. twice daily _____

    c. morning _____

    d. three times daily _____

    e. after meals _____

    f. immediately _____

    g. four times a day _____

    h. while awake _____

    i. every hour _____

    j. night _____

4. Write the word for each of the following measurements.

    a. $\overline{\overline{ss}}$ _____

    b. mL _____

    c. lb _____

    d. kg _____

    e. L _____

Roman Numerals

Write the Roman numerals for each of the following numbers.

1. a. one _____

    b. twelve _____

    c. six _____

    d. nine _____

    e. four _____

2. Unscramble the medical terms and write them in the center of the star. Then define each term in the spaces provided.

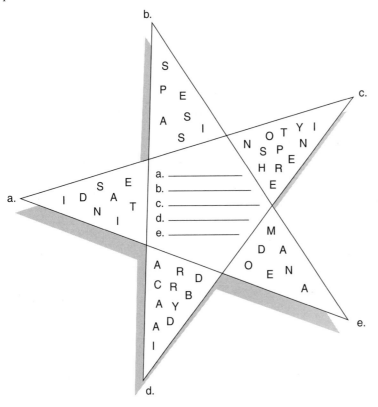

    a. _____

    b. _____

    c. _____

    d. _____

    e. _____

3. Complete the organizational pattern of the body.

    cells → _____ → _____ → systems

4. There are four tissue types. Write their names and list their functions.

    a. _____

    _____

b. _____

_____

c. _____

_____

d. _____

_____

5. Select the proper directional term from the list provided for each area indicated. Then color the organs as specified in the list.

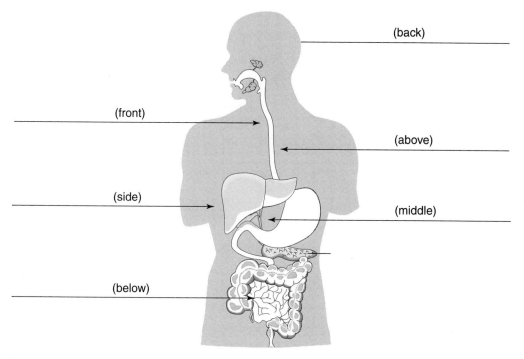

(back)

(front)

(above)

(side)

(middle)

(below)

anterior   medial
inferior   posterior
lateral   superior

Organ Colors

Appendix—brown
Liver—green
Small intestine—red
Pancreas—yellow
Stomach—orange

6. Use the correct term to identify the relationships of the body parts listed by writing the correct answer in the space provided.

Answer

a. breasts	(anterior)	(posterior)	_____
b. heels	(anterior)	(posterior)	_____
c. toes	(anterior)	(posterior)	_____
d. buttocks	(anterior)	(posterior)	_____
e. abdomen	(anterior)	(posterior)	_____
f. breast related to legs	(superior)	(inferior)	_____
g. ankles related to legs	(superior)	(inferior)	_____
h. head related to toes	(superior)	(inferior)	_____
i. hips related to breasts	(superior)	(inferior)	_____
j. thumb related to little finger	(medial)	(lateral)	_____

7. Another term for anterior is _____.

8. Another term for posterior is _____.

9. Write the proper abbreviations for abdominal regions.

   a. Patient A is complaining of pain in the area of his appendix. You properly identify this area as the

   _____.

   b. Patient B is complaining of discomfort in the area of his stomach. You properly identify this area as the

   _____.

   c. Patient C is complaining of pain over the region of his liver. You properly identify this area as the

   _____.

   d. Patient D is complaining of pain over the region where the lower descending colon is located. You properly identify this area as the _____.

Matching

Place the organs in the proper systems.

Organ

1. _____ Spleen
2. _____ Brain
3. _____ Breasts
4. _____ Kidneys
5. _____ Ureters
6. _____ Vagina
7. _____ Bones
8. _____ Heart
9. _____ Pituitary gland
10. _____ Joints

System

a. Cardiovascular
b. Endocrine
c. Digestive
d. Integumentary
e. Skeletal
f. Muscular
g. Nervous
h. Reproductive
i. Respiratory
j. Urinary

Match the function and the system.

Function

1. _____ Transports, absorbs food
2. _____ Regulates body processes through hormones
3. _____ Fulfills sexual needs
4. _____ Brings in oxygen
5. _____ Forms walls of some organs
6. _____ Eliminates liquid wastes
7. _____ Acts as levers in movement
8. _____ Produces hormones to regulate body functions
9. _____ Carries oxygen and nutrients to cells
10. _____ Coordinates body activities through nervous impulses

System

a. Cardiovascular
b. Endocrine
c. Digestive
d. Integumentary
e. Skeletal
f. Muscular
g. Nervous
h. Reproductive
i. Respiratory
j. Urinary

DEVELOPING GREATER INSIGHT

1. With a partner, find the approximate location of the following organs.

   a. brain

   b. heart

   c. lung

   d. stomach

   e. liver

   f. appendix

2. Have a partner indicate pain in some part of his or her body and then describe the area using proper anatomic terms.

3. If available, examine models such as a skeleton or torso or wall chart. Practice naming the major bones and organs.

Classification of Disease

After completing this unit, you will be able to:

- Spell and define terms.
- Define disease and list some possible causes.
- Distinguish between signs and symptoms.
- List six major health problems.
- Identify disease-related terms.
- List ways in which a diagnosis is made.
- Describe malignant and benign tumors.

UNIT SUMMARY

Disease is any change from a healthy state. Disease takes many forms and has many causes. A variety of factors influence promotion of or resistance to disease. Specific terms are used when discussing disease, such as:

- Etiology
- Signs and symptoms
- Prognosis
- Risk factors
- Predisposing factors

Major disease conditions include:

- Congenital disorders
- Traumas
- Chemical imbalances
- Infections
- Ischemias
- Neoplasms

Diagnoses are made using laboratory and other diagnostic tests, including:

- Ultrasound
- Thermography
- Magnetic resonance imaging (MRI)
- X-rays
- Recording of electrical activity of organs
- Direct visualization procedures
- Dye studies
- Cardiac catheterization

Neoplasms are common to body organs. They are:

- Benign or malignant
- Of unknown etiology
- Named as:
  - organ plus *oma* (benign)

◦ sarcomas (malignant)

◦ carcinomas (malignant)

◦ special names

Types of therapy include:

• Surgery

• Chemotherapy

• Radiation

• Supportive care

Body defenses include:

• Unbroken skin

• Mucous membranes

• Mucus

• Acidity of secretions

• White blood cells

• Inflammation

• Immune response

NURSING ASSISTANT ALERT

Action

Observe signs and symptoms carefully.

Report observations promptly.

Benefit

Accurate information is gathered.

Prompt and proper action can be taken.

ACTIVITIES

Vocabulary Exercise

Complete the puzzle by filling in the missing letters of words found in this unit. Use the definitions to help you discover these words.

1. naming the disease process
2. protective body chemicals
3. seen by others
4. abnormalities present at birth
5. injury
6. new growth
7. treatment
8. Define disease.

1.   D _ _ _ _ _ _ _
2. _ _ _ _ _ _ _ I _ _
3.   S _ _ _ _
4. _ _ _ _ E _ _ _ _
5.   _ _ A _ _ _
6. _ _ _ _ _ _ S _
7.   _ _ E _ _ _ _

9. Define etiology.

Matching

Match each clinical condition with the proper pathological classification.

Condition

1. _____ fractured femur
2. _____ pneumonia
3. _____ spina bifida
4. _____ rectal abscess
5. _____ diabetes
6. _____ lupus erythematosis
7. _____ osteoma
8. _____ thrombosis

Classification

a. ischemia
b. congenital abnormality
c. infection
d. neoplasia
e. trauma
f. inflammation
g. metabolic imbalance
h. obstruction
i. autoimmune reaction

Match the clinical condition with the common cause or predisposing factor.

Condition

9. _____ trauma
10. _____ age
11. _____ malnutrition
12. _____ tumors
13. _____ microorganisms
14. _____ radiation
15. _____ heredity

Classification

a. external
b. internal
c. predisposing

Condition

16. _____ radiation
17. _____ rash
18. _____ nausea
19. _____ pain
20. _____ elevated temperature
21. _____ increased pulse rate
22. _____ vomiting
23. _____ flushed skin
24. _____ dizziness
25. _____ itching
26. _____ anxious feelingss

Classification

a. sign
b. symptom

Completion

Complete the statements in the spaces provided.

1. You are assigned to the pediatric unit and have five patients in your care. Briefly explain each of their diagnoses.

   a. Jessica R has hemophilia.

   _____

   b. Billy B has sickle cell anemia.

   _____

   c. Jennifer F has talipes.

   _____

d. Casey B has cleft lip.

_____

e. Leslie S has renal agenesis.

_____

2. Each of these cases falls into the classification of disease known as
_____ or _____.

3. The following week you are working in a surgical unit and find these names and diagnoses on your assignment. Define each diagnosis.

a. Mrs. McFarland—nephroptosis

_____

b. Ms. Horton—cholelithiasis

_____

c. Mr. Hughes—renal lithiasis

_____

d. Mrs. Ramirez—cerebral thrombosis

_____

4. The conditions in the previous question involve _____ to the flow of body fluids.

5. Several of your other patients have diagnoses of metabolic imbalances. List four conditions you have learned that fall into this classification.

a. _____

b. _____

c. _____

d. _____

6. One of your patients has been admitted for surgery with a diagnosis of adenoma.
You recognize this as a _____ involving a _____.

7. Mrs. Bolen has been admitted for tests because of a possible diagnosis of cancer. List six signs and symptoms of cancer you might note when caring for her.

a. _____

b. _____

c. _____

d. _____

e. _____

f. _____

8. The body has special natural defenses. List five.

a. _____

b. _____

c. _____

d. _____

e. _____

9. List four basic forms of therapy.

   a. _____

   b. _____

   c. _____

   d. _____

Clinical Situations

Briefly describe how a nursing assistant should react to each of the following situations.

1. Your neighbor Elizabeth Simmons tells you she has a lump in her breast but she has told no one else.

   _____

   _____

   _____

2. Mrs. Torres has a cerebral thrombus. Follow the maze to identify its location.

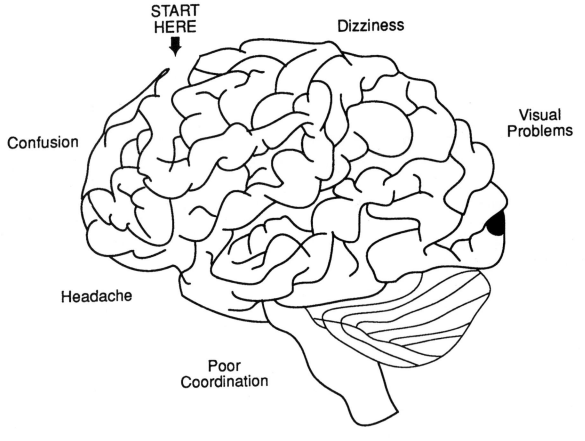

   a. What part of the body is affected? _____

   b. Define the words:

      cerebral _____

      thrombus _____

DEVELOPING GREATER INSIGHT

1. Discuss the importance of mammograms with the class. Invite anyone who has had a mammogram to share her impressions of the experience, or ask a technician to discuss the procedure.

2. Review an unidentified case history of a person who suffered a stroke. Try to relate what you are hearing about the case to the material you have learned in this unit.

3. Discuss the use of ultrasound and MRI as diagnostic tools. Invite anyone who has undergone one of these tests to discuss their experience, or ask a technician to discuss the procedures.

Basic Human Needs and Communication

U N I T **7**

Communication Skills

OBJECTIVES

After completing this unit, you will be able to:

- Spell and define terms.
- Explain the types of verbal and nonverbal communication.
- Describe and demonstrate how to answer the telephone while on duty.
- Describe four tools of communication for staff members.
- Describe the guidelines for communicating with patients with impaired hearing, impaired vision, aphasia, and disorientation.
- State the guidelines for working with interpreters.

UNIT SUMMARY

Communication is a two-way process of sharing information. Communications must be clear between yourself and patients, co-workers, and those in authority. Communications are sent through:

- Oral or verbal language
- Body language
- Written messages

Special communication techniques must be used when communicating with patients who have aphasia, who have impaired hearing or vision, or who are disoriented.

NURSING ASSISTANT ALERT

Action	Benefit
Communicate effectively with co-workers.	Ensures that accurate information is transmitted properly. Ensures that the safest care will be given.
Communicate effectively with patients.	Ensures that patients' needs will be recognized and understood. Means that patients will properly understand directions.
Communicate effectively with families and visitors.	Conveys a feeling of welcome and security to family members and visitors.

ACTIVITIES

Vocabulary Exercise

Define the following by selecting the correct term from the list provided.

aphasia

communication

memo

eye contact

symbols

body language

disorientation

nonverbal communication

sign language

verbal communication

1. Objects used to represent something else _____

2. A state of mental confusion _____

3. Spoken words _____

4. Inability to understand spoken or written language, or inability to express spoken or written language _____

5. Makes the greatest impression during communication and will be remembered the longest _____

6. Communicating through body movements _____

7. Form of communication used by some persons with hearing impairment _____

8. Communicating without oral speech _____

9. Brief written communication that informs or reminds employees _____

10. Exchanging information _____

Completion

Complete the statements in the spaces provided.

1. Describe the purpose of each of the following.

   a. Employee's personnel handbook

   _____

b. Disaster manual

_____

c. Procedure manual

_____

d. Nursing policy manual

_____

e. Assignment

_____

2. List types of information that might be learned in a staff development class.

a. _____

b. _____

c. _____

d. _____

3. Four things are needed for successful communication. They are:

a. _____

b. _____

c. _____

d. _____

4. List six ways in which people communicate without using words.

a. _____

b. _____

c. _____

d. _____

e. _____

f. _____

5. State five ways you can improve communications with patients.

a. _____

b. _____

c. _____

d. _____

e. _____

6. List three important activities that are part of active listening.

a. _____

b. _____

c. _____

Observation, Reporting, and Documentation

OBJECTIVES

After completing this unit, you will be able to:

- Spell and define terms.
- List the components of the nursing process.
- Explain the responsibilities of the nursing assistant for each component of the nursing process.
- Describe two observations to make for each body system.
- State the purpose of the care plan conference.
- List three times when oral reports are given.
- Describe the information given when reporting.
- State the purpose of the patient's medical record.
- Explain the rules for documentation.
- State the purpose of the HIPAA laws.
- Describe the difference between an electronic medical record (EMR), an electronic patient record (EPR), an electronic health record (EHR), and a personal health record (PHR).
- List at least 10 guidelines for computerized documentation.

UNIT SUMMARY

Patient-focused care is carried out most effectively when communications are accurately passed between co-workers and between caregivers and patients. This is achieved by:

- Following the nursing process.
- Developing an individual care plan for each patient.
- Proper documentation and reporting.

The nursing process has four steps, and nursing assistants make a valuable contribution to each. The four steps are:

- Assessment
- Planning
- Implementation
- Evaluation

NURSING ASSISTANT ALERT

Action	Benefit
Observe carefully and report to nurse.	Alerts nurse to changes in patient's condition so proper care can be given.
Document accurately.	Keeps staff informed of patient's status.
Follow nursing care plan faithfully.	Ensures proper patient-focused care for the individual patient.

ACTIVITIES

Vocabulary Exercise

Each line has four different spellings of a word from this unit. Circle the correctly spelled word.

1. assesment   ascesment   accessment   assessment
2. charing   charting   sharting   chartting
3. process   procese   prosess   processe
4. graphic   grephic   grafic   graffic
5. obsavation   obserbation   observation   observachian
6. communication   comunication   cummunication   communikation
7. planing   planning   planinng   pleanning
8. evaleation   evaloation   evaluation   eveluation

Completion

Complete the following statements in the spaces provided.

1. The four steps of the nursing process and their definitions are:

   Step   **Definition**

   a._____   _____

   b. _____   _____

   c._____   _____

   d. _____   _____

2. What are three types of information you will find on the care plan?

   a. _____

   b. _____

   c. _____

3. The nursing diagnosis is a statement of _____

   _____

4. The nursing diagnosis reflects:

    a. _____

    b. _____

    c. _____

    d. _____

5. The nursing diagnosis provides the foundation for _____.

6. The nurse coordinates assessment with _____

    _____

7. The care plan goals must be _____ in order to know if the plan is successful.

8. The intervention (approach) states:

    a. _____

    b. _____

    c. _____

9. Nursing assistants are responsible for knowing when and _____
   the approach is to be carried out and for implementing the approach _____.

10. The final step in the nursing process is the _____.

11. The nursing assistant is responsible for reporting to the nurse when _____

    _____

12. Critical pathways detail the:

    a. _____

    b. _____

13. The critical pathway lists nursing actions to _____.

Differentiation

Differentiate between signs and symptoms by writing each observation under the proper label in the spaces provided.

Sign	**Symptom**	**Observation**
1. _____	_____	nausea
2. _____	_____	vomiting
3. _____	_____	pain
4. _____	_____	restlessness
5. _____	_____	dizziness
6. _____	_____	cold, clammy skin
7. _____	_____	incontinence
8. _____	_____	elevated blood pressure
9. _____	_____	anxiety
10. _____	_____	cough

Matching

Name the sense used to determine the following information.

1. _____   Body odor   a. eyes

2. _____   Radial pulse   b. ears

3. _____   Wheezing when the patient breathes   c. smell

4. _____   Comments from the patient   d. touch

5. _____   Blood in urine

6. _____   A change in the way a patient walks

7. _____   Warmth of the patient's skin

8. _____   Bruises

9. _____   Lump under the patient's skin

10. _____ The patient crying

Matching

Match the observation on the left with the system on the right to which it most relates.

Observation   **System**

1. _____   curled up in bed   a. circulatory

2. _____   disoriented as to time and place   b. integumentary

3. _____   regular pulse   c. muscular

4. _____   elevated blood pressure   d. skeletal

5. _____   jaundiced skin   e. nervous

6. _____   skin warm to touch   f. respiratory

7. _____   difficulty breathing   g. digestive

8. _____   unable to respond with words   h. endocrine

9. _____   cloudy urine   i. reproductive

10. _____ site of injection hot and red   j. urinary

11. _____ difficulty passing stool

12. _____ belching frequently following a meal

13. _____ vaginal discharge

14. _____ drowsy, not responding well

15. _____ nauseated, vomited small amount of clear fluid

Multiple Choice

Select the one best answer for each of the following.

1. To find information about care to be given to an individual patient, you should consult the:

   a. patient's medical record.

   b. procedure manual.

   c. patient care plan.

   d. nursing policy manual.

2. For the most up-to-date information about the patient's condition, check the:

   a. patient's medical record.

   b. nursing policy manual.

   c. procedure manual.

   d. patient care plan.

3. The patient's medical record:

   a. is not a permanent document.

   b. is a legal document.

   c. is the nurses' responsibility.

   d. may be used only while the patient is in the hospital facility.

4. When you report off duty, your report should include:

   a. details on how your day went.

   b. the care you gave each patient.

   c. comments about patients not in your care.

   d. observations on how well the staff got along.

5. Nursing assistants may document on the:

   a. physician's order sheet.

   b. consultant record.

   c. dietary record.

   d. flow sheet.

6. Charting must:

   a. be about all the patients in one room.

   b. address problems listed in the care plan.

   c. include the wishes of the family.

   d. be documented in subjective terms.

7. When charting:

   a. use objective statements.

   b. use complete sentences.

   c. make up abbreviations to save space.

   d. round off times to the closest hour.

8. Your patient has a kidney condition. You should note:

   a. rate of respirations.

   b. edema.

   c. vaginal drainage.

   d. appetite.

9. Your patient has a digestive problem. You should note:

   a. color of sputum.

   b. orientation to time.

   c. belching.

   d. lumps.

10. Your patient has a heart problem. You should note:

    a. regularity of pulse.

    b. mental status.

    c. nasal drainage.

    d. ability to walk.

Matching

Match the regular time and its equivalent in international time.

Regular Time   **International Time**

1. _____ 12:30 AM   a. 1230

2. _____ 7:15 AM   b. 1915

3. _____ 2:30 PM   c. 0800

4. _____ 8 PM   d. 1430

5. _____ 4:30 PM   e. 2000

                                                            f. 0030

                                                            g. 0715

                                                            h. 1630

Completion

Complete each statement as it relates to charting by selecting the proper word from those provided.

blank	recommendation	background	completely	entry
SBAR	sequence	spell	title	cumulative

1. Fill out new headings _____.

2. The _____ is a review of the circumstances leading up to a situation.

3. Date and time each _____.

4. Chart entries in correct _____.

5. Your _____ is what you think should to be done to correct a problem.

6. _____ each word correctly.

7. Leave no _____ spaces between entries.

8. Give report in _____ format.

9. Sign each entry with your first initial, last name, and _____.

10. _____ information is collected over a period of time.

Short Answer

Fill in brief answers in the spaces provided.

1. Fill in the blanks in the diagram. Explain the difference between nursing diagnosis and medical diagnosis.

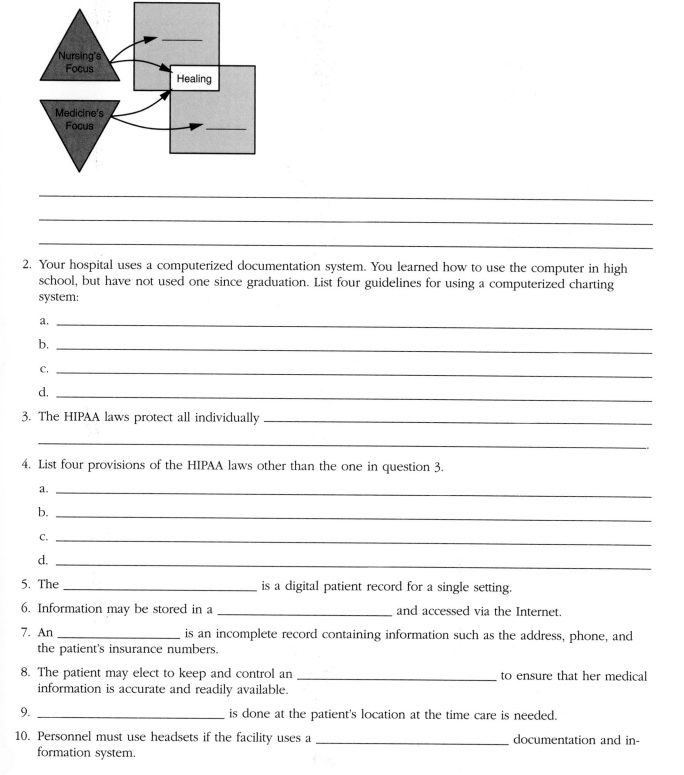

_____

_____

_____

2. Your hospital uses a computerized documentation system. You learned how to use the computer in high school, but have not used one since graduation. List four guidelines for using a computerized charting system:

   a. _____

   b. _____

   c. _____

   d. _____

3. The HIPAA laws protect all individually _____

   _____.

4. List four provisions of the HIPAA laws other than the one in question 3.

   a. _____

   b. _____

   c. _____

   d. _____

5. The _____ is a digital patient record for a single setting.

6. Information may be stored in a _____ and accessed via the Internet.

7. An _____ is an incomplete record containing information such as the address, phone, and the patient's insurance numbers.

8. The patient may elect to keep and control an _____ to ensure that her medical information is accurate and readily available.

9. _____ is done at the patient's location at the time care is needed.

10. Personnel must use headsets if the facility uses a _____ documentation and information system.

Clinical Situations

Answer the following questions in regard to this patient's care.

Robert Gonzales is 62 years of age. He has had a brain attack. He shows right-side weakness, alteration in cerebral tissue perfusion, and aphasia. The nurse has instructed you to assist with all ADLs. The patient showers. Vital signs are to be checked T.I.D.

1. How many times each day will you measure the patient's vital signs?

    _____

2. What kind of help might this patient need in ADLs?

    _____

3. What particular safety measure must you take during the shower?

    _____

4. What problem does the aphasia cause?

    _____

5. Explain the meanings of the following conditions.

    a. right-side weakness _____

    _____

    b. alteration in cerebral tissue perfusion _____

    _____

6. Will raising your voice help Mr. Gonzales understand? Why or why not?

    _____

    _____

7. What are two nonverbal communication techniques that speech therapists sometimes use to help a patient with aphasia?

    a. _____

    b. _____

DEVELOPING GREATER INSIGHT

1. Examine some unidentified care plans. Try giving an oral report based on the information.

2. Select a partner. Using your senses to make observations, then describe the signs or symptoms you identify.

3. Using the unidentified care plans, document the nursing assistant care that is to be given on your shift on facility flow sheets.

UNIT **9**

Meeting Basic Human Needs

OBJECTIVES

After completing this unit, you will be able to:

- Spell and define terms.
- Describe the stages of human growth and development.
- Explain how the generation in which one is born affects the lives of its members.
- List five physical needs of patients.
- Define self-esteem.
- Describe how the nursing assistant can meet the patient's emotional needs.
- List nursing assistant actions to ensure that patients have the opportunity for intimacy.
- Explain why cultural and spiritual beliefs influence patients' psychological responses.
- Discuss methods of dealing with the fearful patient.
- List the guidelines to assist patients in meeting their spiritual needs.

UNIT SUMMARY

Individuals develop at varying rates. There are, however, some well-defined developmental stages through which each person passes.

- Certain developmental skills are characteristically acquired at certain stages of life—from birth to death. A person's success in mastering these skills affects the progress of his development.
- Regardless of developmental level, people have common basic emotional and physical needs.

- The nursing staff must be sensitive to the influence of culture on the expression of individual needs.
- The way in which these needs are expressed varies, especially when a person is ill.
- The nursing staff must be sensitive to patients' individual needs. They must find ways of successfully providing for them.

53

NURSING ASSISTANT ALERT

Action

Recognize that age groups differ in levels of development.

Accept people as unique individuals with basic needs.

Recognize that personal preferences for care, food, clothing, music, activities, and so forth are all affected by the patients' age, generation, and culture.

Benefit

Each patient will be treated as an individual.

Care plans will be developed that consider and meet personal needs.

Treat all patients in an age-appropriate manner.

ACTIVITIES

Vocabulary Exercise

Unscramble the words introduced in this unit and define them. Select terms from the list provided.

continuum	growth	preadolescence	development
intimacy	sexuality	reflex	neonate
toddler	generation	transgender	adolescence

1. T E N O A N E _____
2. C E C A E N R E L D O P E S _____
3. I T R E A G E N O N _____
4. N U C T O I N M U _____
5. L D O T D R E _____
6. W G O R H T _____
7. E E E A C C O D L S N _____
8. P O N L E E V D T E M _____
9. T I M A C I N Y _____
10. D A E N N E R S R G T _____
11. X E F E L R _____
12. U X A L I T S E Y _____

Matching

1. In the playroom for ambulatory patients, you find six children to check. Indicate which children are demonstrating behavior appropriate for their age group by marking A for appropriate or I for inappropriate.

   a. _____ Scott, 16, is receiving an IV and is talking to Patty, 17, who is 2 days postoperative following an appendectomy.

   b. _____ Bobbi, age 13, is stringing beads to make a bracelet.

c. _____ Felicia, age 8, and Kimmie, 11, are playing Pokémon Monopoly.

d. _____ Tommy, 14, and Brian, 15, are playing with the wooden cars and trucks.

e. _____ Johnny, 2½, is playing with blocks near the older boys.

f. _____ Doña, age 3, is sitting near Joanie, pushing different-shaped blocks through the precut holes in a plastic ball.

2. Match the proper term on the right with the explanation of sexual expression on the left.

a. _____ sexual attraction to members of both sexes

b. _____ self-stimulation for sexual pleasure

c. _____ sexual attraction between members of the same sex

d. _____ sexual attraction to members of the opposite sex

1. masturbation

2. homosexuality

3. bisexuality

4. heterosexuality

Completion

Complete the statements in the spaces provided.

1. The stages of growth and development refer to the _____ that must be mastered before moving on to the next stage.

2. Jimmy Hinkle is 12 months old. He weighs 16 pounds and is 26 inches tall. You know this is _____ than average for his chronological age.

3. The average vocabulary of a 2-year-old is about _____ words.

4. Members of each generation are affected by the same _____.

5. Five characteristics of early adulthood include:

a. _____

b. _____

c. _____

d. _____

e. _____

6. The sandwich generation of middle age refers to _____

_____.

7. The time that elapses between the birth of a set of parents and the birth of their offspring is a _____

_____.

8. Later maturity is characterized by a period of _____

_____.

9. The first U.S. generation to be given a label was the _____

_____.

Short Answer

Briefly answer the following questions or directions.

1. Explain Erickson's belief regarding personality development.

_____

_____

2. Briefly explain Maslow's theory regarding human needs.

_____

_____

_____

3. Complete the chart.

STAGES OF GROWTH AND DEVELOPMENT

Neonate	Birth to 1 month
Infancy	a.
b.	2 years to 3 years
Preschool	3 years to 5 years
School Age	5 years to 12 years
Preadolescence	c.
Adolescence	14 years to 20 years
d.	20 years to 49 years
Middle Age	50 years to 64 years
Later Maturity	e.
Old Age	75 years and beyond
f.	Category used by some experts to describe those age 85 and older

TASKS OF PERSONALITY DEVELOPMENT ACCORDING TO THE STAGES DEFINED BY ERIKSON

Physical Stage	Year of Occurrence	Tasks to Be Mastered
Oral-sensory	Birth–1 year (infant)	a.
Muscular-anal	1–3 years (toddler)	b.
Locomotor	3–5 years (preschool years)	To recognize self as a family member (Initiative)
c.	6–11 years (school-age years)	To demonstrate physical and mental skills/abilities (Industry)
Adolescence	12–18 years	d.
e.	19–35 years	To establish intimate personal relationships with a mate (Intimacy)
Adulthood	f.	To live a satisfying and productive life
Maturity	50+ years	g.

Clinical Situations

Briefly explain why you think the patient is acting this way and how you think the nursing assistant should react to the following situations.

1. Jeannie Hunt, age 16, has been diagnosed as suffering from osteosarcoma of her right tibia. The prognosis is guarded and she has been scheduled for surgery to remove the right leg at mid-calf, to be followed by radiation. She asks to see the youth leader of her church.

   _____

   _____

2. Craig Martin, age 52, is recovering from a partial prostatectomy. He is complaining loudly about his care, the food, and the other patients in the room.

   _____

   _____

3. You are serving nourishments and find the door to Rudolph Baker's room closed.

   _____

   _____

4. You are assigned to care for the two male patients in Room 762. You have reason to believe that they may be lovers and another nursing assistant asks you what you know about their relationship.

   _____

   _____

5. Every time you enter Belinda Mitchell's room, she makes sexual advances to you and tries to find reasons to touch you.

   _____

   _____

Relating to the Nursing Process

Write the step of the nursing process that is related to the nursing assistant action.

Nursing Assistant Action	Nursing Process Step
1. The nursing assistant assists the mature adult to ambulate.	_____
2. The nursing assistant reports that the 18-month-old baby has difficulty sitting up.	_____
3. The nursing assistant reports that the teenager still appears to be having periods of depression.	_____
4. The nursing assistant pads the oxygen cannula to reduce irritation behind the patient's ears.	_____
5. The nursing assistant notifies the nurse that Mrs. Tsai has met her care plan goal for bathing two days in a row.	_____
6. The nursing assistant cleans Mr. Hernandez after he was incontinent.	_____
7. The nursing assistant notifies the nurse immediately when she finds that Kelly, age 4, has a rectal temperature of 104°F.	_____
8. The nursing assistant rocks the infant when she cries.	_____

UNIT **10**

Comfort, Pain, Rest, and Sleep

OBJECTIVES

After completing this unit, you will be able to:

- Spell and define terms.
- Explain how noise affects patients and hospital staff.
- Explain why nursing comfort measures are important to patients' well-being.
- List six observations to make and report for patients having pain.
- State the purpose of the pain rating scale and briefly describe how a pain scale is used.
- Describe nursing assistant measures to increase comfort, relieve pain, and promote rest and sleep.
- Describe the phases of the sleep cycle and the importance of each.

UNIT SUMMARY

- Everyone needs comfort, rest, and sleep for physical and emotional well-being, health, and wellness.

- Comfort is a state of physical and emotional well-being. When a patient is comfortable, she is calm and relaxed, and is not in pain or upset.

- Pain is a state of discomfort that is unpleasant. Pain signifies that something is wrong.

- Pain interferes with the patient's level of function and ability to do self-care. It negatively affects quality of life.

- Pain causes stress and anxiety, interfering with comfort, rest, and sleep.

- The patient's self-report of pain is the most accurate indicator of the existence and intensity of pain, and should be reported to the nurse, respected, and believed.

- Patients' complaints of pain always require further intervention.

- Pain rating scales are communication tools that help with assessment and prevent caregivers from forming their own opinions about the level of the patient's pain. Pain scales prevent subjective opinions, provide consistency, eliminate some barriers to pain management, and give the patient a means of describing the pain accurately.

- Rest is a state of mental and physical comfort, calmness, and relaxation. Basic needs of hunger, thirst, elimination, and pain must be met before rest is possible.

- A patient who is resting may sit or lie down, or do things that are pleasant and relaxing.

- Sleep is a basic need that occurs during a period of continuous or intermittent unconsciousness in which physical movements are decreased.

- Adequate sleep is necessary for the body and mind to function properly, and for healing to occur.

- Many factors, both within control and beyond control, affect patients' comfort, rest, and sleep.

- Nonrapid eye movement (NREM) sleep has four phases, progressing from light to very deep.

- Rapid eye movement (REM) sleep restores mental function.

- Care should be scheduled to allow uninterrupted sleep whenever possible.

- A major nursing assistant responsibility is to provide basic personal care and comfort measures to help relieve pain and promote comfort, rest, and sleep.

NURSING ASSISTANT ALERT

Action	Benefit
Ensure privacy, reduce noise, eliminate unpleasant odors, and adjust the temperature, lighting, and ventilation.	Reduces factors that cause discomfort over which the patient has no control.
Handle the patient gently, assist the patient to assume a comfortable position, use pillows and props for repositioning, give a backrub, and provide emotional support.	Helps the patient to relax and rest better. Enhances comfort.
Meet the patient's basic needs of hunger, thirst, elimination, pain relief, and good hygiene.	Relieves factors that interfere with proper rest.
Schedule care to prevent awakening the patient from sleep.	Helps the patient to sleep well, facilitating rest and healing of both mind and body.

ACTIVITIES

Vocabulary Exercise

Complete the crossword puzzle.

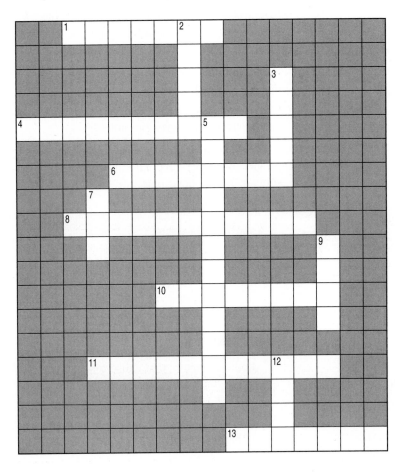

Across

 1 Grinding teeth

 4 A condition in which patients have sudden, uncontrollable, unpredictable urges to fall asleep during the daytime hours

 6 A chronic deprivation of quality or quantity of sleep because sleep is ended or interrupted prematurely

 8 Prolonged sleep loss, or inadequate quality or quantity of sleep

10 Bedwetting

11 A disorder characterized by sleeping very late in the morning and napping during the day

13 A state of physical and emotional well-being in which the patient is calm and relaxed, and is not in pain or upset

Down

2 A basic human need that consists of a period of continuous or intermittent unconsciousness in which physical movements are decreased

3 A potentially serious condition in which breathing stops for 10 seconds or more during sleep

5 Sleepwalking

7 The part of the sleep cycle in which dreams occur

9 A state of mental and physical comfort, calmness, and relaxation

12 The part of the sleep cycle that begins when the patient first falls asleep

Short Answer

Briefly complete the following.

1. List eight factors that may interfere with a patient's ability to sleep.

   a. _____

   b. _____

   c. _____

   d. _____

   e. _____

   f. _____

   g. _____

   h. _____

2. List eight observations that you see, hear, feel, or smell that should be reported to the nurse regarding a patient's pain.

   a. _____

   b. _____

   c. _____

   d. _____

   e. _____

   f. _____

   g. _____

   h. _____

3. How is the patient's outward expression of pain affected by culture?

   _____

4. List at least eight factors that affect patients' comfort, rest, and sleep.

   a. _____

   b. _____

c. _____

d. _____

e. _____

f. _____

g. _____

h. _____

5. What is the purpose of the pain rating scale?

   _____

6. Why is using the pain rating scale a key to consistent pain evaluation?

   _____

7. Why is uninterrupted REM sleep important?

   _____

8. Define the following:

   a. acute pain _____

   b. radiating pain _____

   c. chronic pain _____

   d. phantom pain _____

9. Your patient uses the FACES pain scale. The nurse gave her pain medication an hour ago. The patient tells you that her pain is now number 4. You should:

   _____

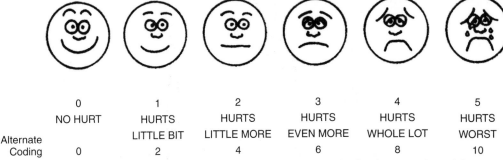

	0 NO HURT	1 HURTS LITTLE BIT	2 HURTS LITTLE MORE	3 HURTS EVEN MORE	4 HURTS WHOLE LOT	5 HURTS WORST
Alternate Coding	0	2	4	6	8	10

(FACES Pain Rating Scale from Hockenberry, M J, Wilson D: Wong's essentials of pediatric nursing, ed. 8. St. Louis 2009, Mosby. Used with permission. Copyright Mosby)

True/False

Mark the following true or false by circling T or F.

1. T   F   The nurse's assessment is always more accurate than a patient's self-report of pain intensity.

2. T   F   A patient must be lying in bed to rest properly.

3. T   F   Comfort is a state of well-being.

4. T   F   A patient with somnambulism is at high risk of injury during sleep.

5. T F   Full-color dreams occur during the NREM phase of the sleep cycle.

6. T F   Elderly adults require about 5 to 7 hours of sleep per day.

7. T F   Toddlers require 12 to 14 hours of sleep a day.

8. T F   Phantom pain is psychological pain.

9. T F   The body repairs itself during sleep.

10. T F   A patient who is resting may pray or say the rosary.

11. T F   Hunger and thirst do not interfere with the ability to rest when a person is sick.

12. T F   Lack of privacy may affect the patient's comfort and ability to rest.

13. T F   There are two phases of the NREM sleep cycle.

14. T F   The patient passes into REM sleep within approximately 60 to 90 minutes after falling asleep.

15. T F   Hypersomnia is a chronic deprivation of quality or quantity of sleep because sleep is ended or interrupted prematurely.

16. T F   According to the EPA, hospital noises should not exceed 138 decibels during the day.

17. T F   Some patients regard excessive noise as an invasion of their privacy.

18. T F   Excessive noise has no effect on the stress level of staff.

19. T F   Hospital workers must be active listeners for good communication.

20. T F   Body language is not affected by pain.

21. T F   A confused patient with garbled speech may be able to describe her pain accurately.

22. T F   Because nurses assess pain, the nursing assistant need not bother learning about the pain scales the facility uses.

23. T F   Unrelieved pain affects the patient's health.

24. T F   Unrelieved pain may cause feelings of anxiety.

Relating to the Nursing Process

1. List 10 things the nursing assistant can do to enhance comfort, rest, and sleep and relieve pain.

    a. _____

    b. _____

    c. _____

    d. _____

    e. _____

    f. _____

    g. _____

    h. _____

    i. _____

    j. _____

DEVELOPING GREATER INSIGHT

1. Your patient, Mrs. Hernandez, has spinal stenosis and frequently complains of pain. The nurse alternates an injection for pain with an oral medication every 2 hours.

   a. Mrs. Hernandez is laughing and visiting with her family. When you enter the room with fresh ice water, she tells you she is in pain. Can a patient who is laughing and visiting be having pain? Explain your answer.

   _____

   _____

   _____

   _____

   _____

   b. Mrs. Hernandez refuses her supper tray. She tells you she is in too much pain to eat. What action should you take?

   _____

   _____

   _____

   _____

   _____

   c. Mrs. Hernandez tells you she feels better now, and would like to eat. The kitchen has closed for the evening. What action should you take?

   _____

   _____

   _____

   _____

   _____

   d. Why do you think that hunger, thirst, pain, and need to use the bathroom affect patients' comfort and ability to rest or sleep?

   _____

   _____

   _____

   _____

   _____

   e. Mrs. Hernandez cannot sleep. She tells you that her low back really hurts. What nursing assistant measures can you take to make her more comfortable?

   _____

   _____

   _____

   _____

   _____

Developing Cultural Sensitivity

OBJECTIVES

After completing this unit, you will be able to:

- Spell and define terms.
- Name six major cultural groups in the United States.
- Describe ways the major cultures differ in their family organization, need for personal space, communication, health practices, religions, and traditions.
- List ways nursing assistants can develop sensitivity about cultures other than their own.
- List ways the nursing assistant can help patients in practicing rituals appropriate to their cultures.
- State ways the nursing assistant can demonstrate appreciation of and sensitivity to other cultures.

UNIT SUMMARY

Patients have a variety of cultural heritages. These heritages influence how individuals:

- Communicate.
- React to health concerns.
- View one another and the need for personal space.
- Celebrate holidays.
- Select foods.
- Express and practice religious beliefs.

Culture also may affect:

- The patient's beliefs about health, wellness, and illness.
- How the patient reacts to illness.
- The patient's hygienic practices.
- The patient's expectations about how care should be given and by whom.
- The patient's participation in self-care during times of illness.

Six ethnic groups predominate in the United States:

- Caucasian
- African American
- Hispanic
- Asian/Pacific
- Native American
- Middle Eastern/Arab

Nursing assistants must treat all patients as individuals and be sensitive to:

- The patient's acceptance of caregivers.
- The amount of disrobing permitted.
- The degree of touch that is comfortable.

NURSING ASSISTANT ALERT

Action

Learn as much as possible about a patient's culture.

Treat patients as individuals within a culture.

Be sensitive to patients' needs relating to personal space, touching, and religious practices.

Benefit

Helps patients receive more personalized care.

Assures that care will be personalized.

Increases patient's sense of acceptance and respect.

ACTIVITIES

Vocabulary Exercise

Complete the puzzle by filling in the missing letters. Use the definitions to help you discover the words.

```
              P
1. _ _ _ _ E _ _ _ _ _ _
              R
2. _ _ _ _ S _ _ _ _
              O
3.    _ _ _ N _ _ _ _ _
              A
4.    _ _ _ L _ _
5.    _ _ _ S _ _ _ _ _ _
              P
6.        _ A _ _
              C
7.    _ _ _ E _
```

Definitions

1. Beliefs that are rigid and based on generalizations
2. Engraved objects used to ward off evil
3. Special group within a race as defined by national origin/culture
4. Charm against evil
5. Ability to be aware of and to appreciate personal characteristics of others
6. Classification of people according to shared physical characteristics
7. Customs

Short Answer

Briefly answer the following questions.

1. What are the six major ethnic groups in the United States?

    a. _____

    b. _____

    c. _____

    d. _____

    e. _____

    f. _____

2. What is meant by "cross-cultural" nursing?

    _____

    _____

3. What effect does living in a new culture have on the cultural values and traditions of the country of origin?

    _____

    _____

    _____

4. People are classified as a race according to which shared physical characteristics?

    _____

    _____

    _____

5. What features do members of ethnic groups have in common?

    _____

    _____

    _____

    _____

6. What are five cultural differences between ethnic groups?

    a. _____

    b. _____

    c. _____

    d. _____

    e. _____

7. What are three beliefs shared by members of a culture?

    a. _____

    b. _____

    c. _____

8. What are the five major religions in the United States?

    a. _____

b. _____

c. _____

d. _____

e. _____

True/False

Mark the following true or false by circling T or F.

1. T   F   Family organization determines who is responsible for making health care decisions.

2. T   F   In Caucasian families, the father is the dominant decision maker.

3. T   F   In extended families, caregiving and personal care are shared responsibilities.

4. T   F   A nuclear family usually includes aunts, uncles, and grandparents.

5. T   F   African Americans prefer to stand far away (more than 3 feet) when speaking with others.

6. T   F   Asians consider direct eye contact inappropriate.

7. T   F   Prolonged eye contact is considered disrespectful by Hispanics.

8. T   F   It is proper for only men to shake hands in Middle Eastern countries.

9. T   F   Uncovering the shoulders of a person from India may be considered disrespectful.

10. T   F   People who are bilingual may revert to their language of origin when under stress.

11. T   F   Dialects may vary between different groups that share a common culture.

RELATING TO THE NURSING PROCESS

Write the step of the nursing process that is related to the nursing assistant action.

Nursing Assistant Action	Nursing Process Step
1. The nursing assistant reports her observations that the patient cannot speak and understand English easily.	_____
2. The nursing assistant stands at a distance that is comfortable for the patient when giving care.	_____
3. The nursing assistant asks politely about practices that are unfamiliar.	_____
4. The nursing assistant provides privacy when a spiritual advisor visits.	_____

DEVELOPING GREATER INSIGHT

1. Your patient, Mr. Dang, is 82 and has lived in this country for several years. He was born in Vietnam, is a Buddhist, and is bilingual.

   a. Of what major ethnic group is Mr. Dang a member?

   _____

b. How might he view the cause of his illness?

_____

c. What part of his care do you think his family might feel responsible for?

_____

d. What deity would Mr. Dang worship?

_____

e. As a culture, how do Asian Americans feel about direct eye contact?

_____

f. Why would it be unwise to stereotype this person?

_____

2. Your patient, Ms. Ruiz, is 76. Her leg was fractured in several places when she was hit by a car. She is in balanced traction on your unit. She is originally from Costa Rica and speaks Spanish with limited English. She tells you that she is being punished for past sins. She wants to see a *curandera*.

a. How might you improve your ability to communicate with her?

_____

_____

b. What four religious articles might be important to her?

_____

_____

c. In what religious ceremony might she wish to participate?

_____

_____

3. List some family practices, events, or celebrations related to your ethnicity.

_____

_____

_____

4. America is a nation of immigrants. Unless you are Native American, your ancestors came from other countries. List as many countries as you can. Provide as much information about each person as possible. Be prepared to discuss it in class. For example: Great grandfather-Scotland-wore a kilt and played drums in a Scottish band. Came to the US in 1893.

Infection and Infection Control

Infection

OBJECTIVES

After completing this unit, you will be able to:

- Spell and define terms.
- Identify the most common microbes and describe some of their characteristics.
- List the links in the chain of infection.
- List the ways in which infectious diseases are spread.
- Name and briefly describe five serious infectious diseases.
- Identify the causes of several important infectious diseases.
- Define spores and explain how spores differ from other pathogens.
- Describe common treatments for infectious disease.
- List natural body defenses against infections.
- Explain why patients are at risk for infections.

UNIT SUMMARY

Pathogens are microscopic organisms that cause disease. Pathogens differ from one another in the way they:

- Look.
- Cause disease.
- Grow.

Pathogens:

- Enter and leave the body by special routes known as *portals of entry* and *portals of exit*.
- Transmit disease by direct and indirect means.
- May be kept alive in reservoirs.

6. Give five examples of fomites found in the health care facility.

a. _____

b. _____

c. _____

d. _____

e. _____

RELATING TO THE NURSING PROCESS

Nursing Assistant Action   **Nursing Process Step**

1. The nursing assistant reports an elevation of
   Mr. Bergen's temperature and redness near
   his infusion site.   _____

2. The nursing assistant makes sure that Mr. Popejoy,
   who has pneumonia, has plenty of tissues and
   a place to dispose of them.   _____

3. The nursing assistant reports that Mr. Menendez
   is coughing frequently as he is admitted.   _____

DEVELOPING GREATER INSIGHT

Match the action with the related portion of the chain of infection.

1. _____ receiving antibiotics when infected   a. protecting the portal of entry

2. _____ disinfecting bedpans   b. protecting the portal of exit

3. _____ covering a draining pressure ulcer   c. protecting a susceptible host

4. _____ not coming to work when you have a cold   d. controlling the causative agents

5. _____ putting a Band-Aid over a cut in your skin   e. eliminating the reservoir

6. Discuss with the class the value of immunization procedures. Try to answer the following:

   a. Which vaccines are commonly given?

   b. When should vaccines be given?

   c. How do vaccines offer protection?

   d. Are there some infections for which there are no immunizations?

Infection Control

After completing this unit, you will be able to:

- Spell and define terms.
- Explain the principles of medical asepsis.
- State the purpose of standard precautions.
- List the types of personal protective equipment.
- Describe nursing assistant actions related to standard precautions.
- Describe airborne, droplet, and contact precautions.
- Demonstrate the following procedures:

Procedure 1	Handwashing
Procedure 2	Putting on a Mask
Procedure 3	Putting on a Gown
Procedure 4	Putting on Gloves
Procedure 5	Removing Contaminated Gloves
Procedure 6	Removing Contaminated Gloves, Eye Protection, Gown, and Mask
Procedure 7	Serving a Meal in an Isolation Unit
Procedure 8	Measuring Vital Signs in an Isolation Unit
Procedure 9	Transferring Nondisposable Equipment Outside of the Isolation Unit
Procedure 10	Specimen Collection from a Patient in an Isolation Unit
Procedure 11	Caring for Linens in an Isolation Unit
Procedure 12	Transporting a Patient to and from the Isolation Unit
Procedure 13	Opening a Sterile Package

UNIT SUMMARY

When patients have communicable diseases that are easily transmitted to others, special procedures must be used. The patient is placed in isolation. Everyone who comes into contact with the patient must practice appropriate isolation techniques. The emphasis is on the infectious material that carries the specific micro-organisms. The goal of the health care provider is to interrupt the chain of infection by preventing transmission of the microbes. By working toward this goal, the health care provider protects the patient, the environment, and self.

The spread of disease can be controlled by:

- Conscientious handwashing.
- Proper medical and surgical asepsis.
- Understanding and faithfully following:
  - Standard precautions.
  - Transmission-based precautions.
  - Isolation techniques.
  - Disinfection and sterilization procedures.

NURSING ASSISTANT ALERT

Action	Benefit
Follow standard precautions exactly.	Prevents transfer of infectious materials.
Give extra attention to isolation patients.	Prevents patient from feeling abandoned.
Place sharps in proper container.	Decreases the danger of sticks or injuries from needles or sharps.
Follow specific transmission-based precautions as outlined in the care plan.	Eliminates unnecessary actions while ensuring that specific transmission prevention techniques are used.
Follow aseptic techniques carefully and accurately.	Protects patients and health care providers from infection.

ACTIVITIES

Vocabulary Exercise

Match the proper term on the right with the definition on the left.

1. Spreads long distances in the air on dust and moisture
2. Centers for Disease Control and Prevention
3. An infectious disease easily transmitted to others
4. Protective hand coverings
5. Expendable
6. Separate ill patients from others
7. Entryway to AIIR room
8. Eye protection that is always worn with a mask
9. One type of mask used in airborne precautions
10. Human immunodeficiency virus
11. _____ pressure air flow is used in an airborne precautions room
12. Contaminated
13. _____ precautions are used any time contact with blood, body fluid, secretions, excretions, mucous membranes, or nonintact skin is likely
14. PPE that covers the uniform

a. anteroom
b. disposable
c. HIV
d. CDC
e. standard
f. HEPA
g. dirty
h. droplet
i. communicable
j. gloves
k. gown
l. isolate
m. goggles

True/False

Mark the following true or false by circling T or F.

1. T   F   Linen found on a linen cart is considered clean.

2. T   F   Linen that has touched the floor is clean as long as the floor is not wet.

3. T   F   Medical aseptic techniques destroy all organisms on an article.

4. T   F   One patient's articles may be used by another as long as the first patient does not have a communicable disease.

5. T   F   Handwashing is not necessary if gloves were worn during patient care.

6. T   F   You can safely touch environmental surfaces with used gloves as long as the gloves are not contaminated with blood.

7. T   F   The nursing assistant is responsible for understanding the principles of standard precautions and selecting personal protective equipment appropriate to the procedure.

8. T   F   Wash your gloves promptly if they become soiled.

9. T   F   Artificial nails are usually acceptable for health care workers as long as they have been professionally applied.

10. T   F   The housekeeping cart and the clean linen cart should be positioned close to each other in the hallway.

11. T   F   Personal medical asepsis includes a daily bath.

12. T   F   Complete personal protective equipment is required when working with all patients.

When washing hands correctly

13. T   F   Always use cool water.

14. T   F   Lean against the sink so no water will get on the floor.

15. T   F   A soap dispenser is preferable to a bar of soap.

16. T   F   Always rinse the bar of soap (if used) after use.

17. T   F   Turn faucets on and off with gloves.

18. T   F   Always point fingertips up when washing.

19. T   F   It is the use of soap that actually removes microbes from hands.

20. T   F   Hands can be washed effectively in 5 to 10 seconds.

21. T   F   Alcohol-based gel may be used instead of handwashing, unless the hands are visibly soiled.

22. T   F   When using an alcohol-based hand cleaner, rub the product into all surfaces for at least 15 seconds.

Completion

Complete the statements in the spaces provided.

1. The purpose of transmission-based precautions is _____

_____

2. Apply a _____when you enter a droplet precautions room.

3. Isolation is the responsibility of _____.

4. The purpose of wearing a mask and gown in the isolation unit is to _____

_____

5. Gloves should be used whenever there may be contact with _____

_____

6. To be effective, a mask must cover both _____ and _____.

7. To be effective, a gown should _____ correctly.

8. The contaminated gown should be folded _____ before you dispose of it in the proper receptacle.

9. Disposable equipment is used only _____.

10. List seven secretions or excretions that are potentially infectious.

    a. _____

    b. _____

    c. _____

    d. _____

    e. _____

    f. _____

    g. _____

11. Breaks in the skin of a health care worker should be immediately treated by _____ and applying

_____.

12. What must be done before these items are used?

    stethoscope   bathtub

    shower chair   wheelchair

_____

Short Answer

1. State the type of infection control that is used in all situations in which care providers may contact body fluids. _____

2. List the three types of transmission-based precautions.

    a. _____

    b. _____

    c. _____

3. List three ways communicable diseases may be spread.

    a. _____

    b. _____

    c. _____

4. List six articles to be placed on a cart outside an isolation room.

    a. _____

    b. _____

    c. _____

    d. _____

    e. _____

    f. _____

5. State the sequence for applying personal protective equipment.

    a. _____

    b. _____

    c. _____

    d. _____

6. List seven precautions to keep in mind when handling soiled linen.

    a. _____

    b. _____

    c. _____

    d. _____

    e. _____

    f. _____

    g. _____

7. State the measures that are to be taken to care for vital sign equipment used with the patient in isolation.

    a. _____

    b. _____

8. Explain what to do with food not eaten by a patient in isolation. _____
_____

9. Name the type of bag that is used for the transport of specimens. _____
_____

10. Name two ways of sterilizing an item.

    a. _____

    b. _____

11. List three respiratory hygiene/cough etiquette practices that patients should be instructed to follow to prevent the spread of infection.

    _____

    _____

    _____

12. UVGI:

    a. Uses _____ light in the _____ or _____.

    b. The purpose of UVGI is to _____.

    c. Does the UVGI light remain on 24 hours a day? _____

    d. Does the radiation emitted from the bright UVGI harm patients' or staff members' eyes? _____

13. When entering the room of a patient who is in isolation for chickenpox, what PPE should you apply?

_____

_____

_____

14. List at least three reasons for wearing gloves. _____

_____

_____

15. List at least five situations when gloves should be worn.

_____

_____

_____

_____

_____

_____

16. Where is PPE removed when leaving the contact precautions room?

_____

_____

17. Where should the respirator be removed when you have finished working in the airborne precautions room?

_____

_____

18. What should be done with the face mask when leaving the room of a patient who is in droplet precautions?

_____

_____

Clinical Situations

Briefly describe how a nursing assistant should react to the following situations.

1. You saw an airborne precautions sign on Mr. Keene's door. You are assigned to serve his breakfast tray.

_____

_____

_____

2. You are responsible for caring for nondisposable equipment from a contact precautions unit.

_____

_____

Identification

1. Identify the sign and indicate the type of precaution to be used.

   a.

   _____

   _____

   b.

   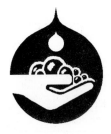

   _____

   _____

   c.

   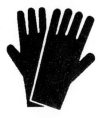

   _____

   _____

d.

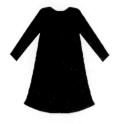

_____

_____

e.

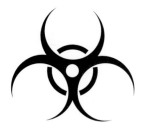

_____

_____

2. Label the diagram of the isolation room.

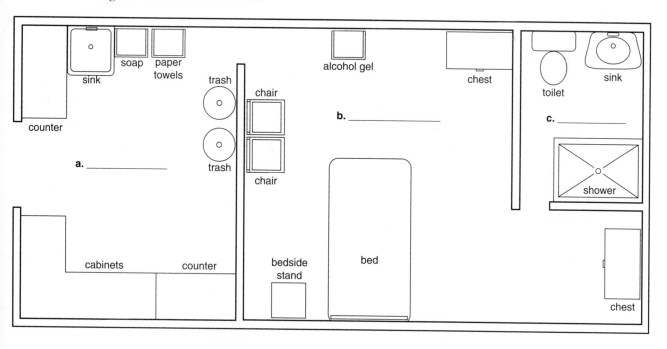

a. _____

b. _____

c. _____

3. Identify what is wrong with each picture. What should be done to correct it?

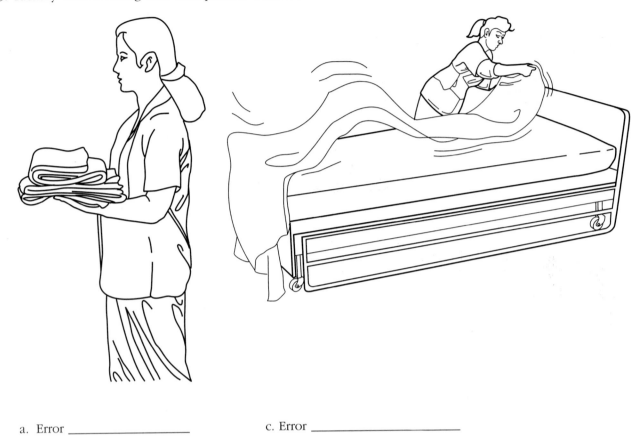

   a. Error _____

   b. Correction _____

      c. Error _____

      d. Correction _____

4. What is wrong with the figure on the left? Correct it in the figure on the right. Use the empty bedside table to demonstrate the correction by locating the articles properly or writing in the words.

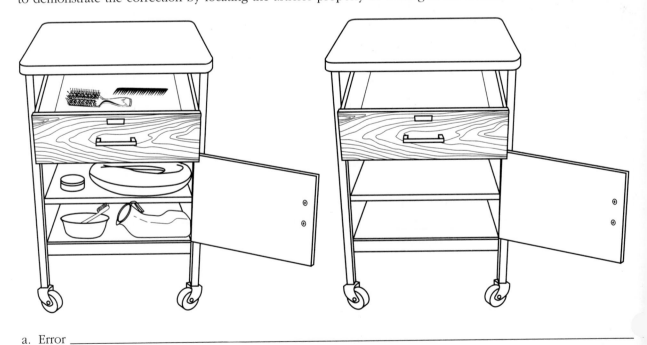

   a. Error _____

   b. Correction _____

5. Briefly explain how the nursing assistant should react to the following. You are assisting the nurse in setting up a sterile field to change a surgical dressing. You open some 4 x 4s and reach across the field and place them on the towel. The nurse tells you the setup cannot be used and must be discarded and set up again. Why?

_____

_____

RELATING TO THE NURSING PROCESS

Write the step of the nursing process that is related to the nursing assistant action.

Nursing Assistant Action   **Nursing Process Step**

1. The nursing assistant is not sure how to transport the patient safely from isolation to the X-ray department, so she asks the team leader for instructions.   _____

2. The nursing assistant carefully removes his contaminated gown and disposes of it properly after completing care in the contact precautions room.   _____

DEVELOPING GREATER INSIGHT

1. With classmates and instructor, explain ways to help patients feel less abandoned when in isolation.

2. Investigate the transmission-based isolation precautions in your facility and report back to the class.

3. Discuss why direct contact with blood and body fluids can be dangerous to a health care worker.

Safety and Mobility

Environmental and Nursing Assistant Safety

OBJECTIVES

After completing this unit, you will be able to:

- Spell and define terms.
- Describe the health care facility environment.
- Identify measures to promote environmental safety.
- List situations when equipment must be repaired.
- Describe the elements required for fire.
- List five measures to prevent a fire.
- Describe the procedure to follow if a fire occurs.
- Demonstrate the use of a fire extinguisher.
- List techniques for using ergonomics on the job.
- Demonstrate appropriate body mechanics.
- Describe the types of information contained in Safety Data Sheets (SDS).

Short Answer

Write the information in the spaces provided.

1. Briefly list seven items you would expect to find in the patient's environment.

   a. _____

   b. _____

   c. _____

   d. _____

   e. _____

   f. _____

   g. _____

2. Name two pieces of fire control equipment.

   a. _____

   b. _____

3. The acronym PASS is important for fire control. The:

   a. P stands for _____.

   b. A stands for _____.

   c. S stands for _____.

   d. S stands for _____.

4. List six ergonomic techniques you can use to decrease the risk of injury.

   a. _____

   b. _____

   c. _____

   d. _____

   e. _____

   f. _____

5. State five types of information you expect to learn from the SDS of a product.

   a. _____

   b. _____

   c. _____

   d. _____

   e. _____

6. List four potential benefits of using side rails.

   a. _____

   b. _____

   c. _____

   d. _____

7. List six potential risks of using side rails.

   a. _____

   b. _____

   c. _____

   d. _____

   e. _____

   f. _____

8. List five areas that are usually equipped with emergency lighting in the event of a power failure.

   a. _____

   b. _____

   c. _____

   d. _____

   e. _____

9. List six methods of preventing a fire.

   a. _____

   b. _____

   c. _____

   d. _____

   e. _____

   f. _____

10. Draw the fire triangle, showing its elements.

Patient Safety and Positioning

OBJECTIVES

After completing this unit, you will be able to:

- Spell and define terms.
- Identify patients who are at risk for having incidents.
- List alternatives to the use of physical restraints.
- Describe the guidelines for the use of restraints.
- Demonstrate the correct application of restraints.
- Describe two measures for preventing accidental poisoning, thermal injuries, skin injuries, and choking.
- List the elements that are common to all procedures.
- Describe correct body alignment for the patient.
- List the purposes of repositioning patients.
- State the purpose of assistive moving devices.
- Demonstrate these positions using the correct supportive devices: supine, semisupine, prone, semiprone, lateral, Fowler's, and orthopneic.
- Demonstrate the following procedures:

    Procedure 14 Turning the Patient Toward You

    Procedure 15 Turning the Patient Away from You

    Procedure 16 Moving a Patient to the Head of the Bed

    Procedure 17 Logrolling the Patient

UNIT SUMMARY

- Take preventive measures to avoid patient incidents.

- Restraints, (if used), must be applied correctly. Follow the care plan and facility restraint policies. Before restraints are used, the staff must assess the patient's capabilities and reasons for use of the restraint. Eliminating the cause of problem behavior may eliminate the need for the restraint.

- Alternatives to restraints should be used whenever possible. If restraints are necessary, the least amount of restraint should be used for the least amount of time necessary to keep the patient safe.

- *Enablers* are devices that empower patients and assist them to function at their highest possible level.

- Side rails are restraints in some circumstances. They are also enablers in some situations.

- Position the patient in good alignment and provide support at all times in all positions.

- Frequent change of position helps prevent deformities and pressure ulcers. It also aids general body functions and contributes to comfort.

- Frequent position changes are essential to prevent:

  ○ Musculoskeletal deformities and loss of calcium from bone.

  ○ Poor skin nutrition and the development of pressure ulcers.

  ○ Severe constipation and fecal impaction.

  ○ Respiratory complications such as pneumonia.

  ○ Decreased circulation that could lead to thrombophlebitis and renal calculi.

  ○ Loss of opportunities for social exchange between patient and staff.

- Procedures list step-by-step directions for giving patient care. Each facility may have slight variations. Become familiar with the procedures used in your facility and follow them faithfully.

- Some steps are common to all procedures. The initial procedure actions and ending procedure actions are listed here.

Initial Procedure Actions

1. Wash your hands or use an alcohol-based hand cleaner.

2. Assemble supplies and equipment and bring them to the patient's room.

3. Knock on the door and identify yourself.

4. Identify the patient according to facility policy. Some facilities identify people with arm bands. Some ask the patient to recite his or her date of birth.

5. Ask visitors to leave the room and advise where they may wait (as desired by the patient).

6. Explain what you are going to do and what is expected of the patient. Answer questions. (Maintain a dialogue with the patient during the procedure, and repeat explanations and instructions as needed.)

7. Provide privacy by closing the door, privacy curtain, and window curtain. (All three should be closed even if the patient is alone in the room.)

8. Wash your hands or use an alcohol-based hand cleaner.

9. Set up supplies and equipment at the bedside. (Use an overbed table, if possible, or other clean area. Cover with a clean underpad, according to nursing judgment, to provide a clean work surface.) Open packages. Position items for convenient reach. Position a container for soiled items so that you do not have to cross over clean items to access it.

10. Wash your hands or use an alcohol-based hand cleaner.

11. Position the patient for the procedure. Support with pillows and props as needed. Place a clean underpad under the area being treated, as needed. Make sure the patient is comfortable and able to maintain the position throughout the procedure.

12. Cover the patient with a bath blanket and drape for modesty. Fold the bath blanket back to expose only the area on which you will be working.

13. Raise the bed to a comfortable working height.

14. Lock the wheels of the bed, stretcher, etc. if used during the procedure.

15. Apply gloves if contact with blood, moist body fluids (except sweat), secretions, excretions, or nonintact skin is likely.

16. Apply a gown if your uniform will have substantial contact with linen or other articles contaminated with blood, moist body fluid (except sweat), secretions, or excretions.

17. Apply a mask and eye protection if splashing of blood or moist body fluids is likely.

18. Lower the side rail on the side where you will be working.

Ending Procedure Actions

1. Remove gloves.

2. Reposition the patient to ensure that he or she is comfortable and in good body alignment.

3. Replace the bed covers, then remove any drapes used. Place used drapes in a plastic bag to discard in trash or soiled linen.

4. Elevate the side rails, if used, before leaving the bedside.

5. Remove other personal protective equipment, if worn, and discard in plastic bag or according to facility policy.

6. Wash your hands or use an alcohol-based hand cleaner.

7. Return the bed to the lowest horizontal position.

8. Open the privacy and window curtains.

9. Position the call signal and needed personal items within reach.

10. Wash your hands or use an alcohol-based hand cleaner.

11. Remove procedural trash and contaminated linen when you leave the room. Discard in appropriate container or location.

12. Inform visitors that they may return to the room.

13. Document the procedure, your observations, and the patient's response.

   Note: When there are open lesions, wet linen, or possible contact with patient body fluids, blood, secretions, excretions, mucous membranes, or nonintact skin, disposable gloves are to be worn during the procedure. Put on gloves before contact with the patient or linen. Dispose of gloves according to facility policy after removing them. **Always apply standard precautions.**

• Special procedures in this unit relate to positioning, supporting, and restraining patients in a safe, appropriate manner, using proper body mechanics.

NURSING ASSISTANT ALERT

Action	Benefit
Use proper posture and body mechanics during all activities.	Enables the body to function at its best.
Follow the eight basic rules for effective body use.	Prevents injury and reduces fatigue.
Support patients in proper alignment in all positions.	Improves comfort and relieves strain. Prevents deformities. Allows the body to function more effectively.
Apply restraints and supports according to established protocol.	Ensures proper standard of patient care.

ACTIVITIES

Vocabulary Exercise

Complete the puzzle by filling in the missing letters of words found in this unit. Use the definitions to help you discover these words.

1.	__ P __ __ __ __	1. Involving muscle contractions
2.	__ __ __ __ O __ __ __	2. Devices for maintaining the position of extremities
3.	__ __ S __ __ __ __ __	3. Device that inhibits patient movement
4.	__ __ __ __ __ I __ __	4. Ability to move
5.	__ __ __ T __ __ __ __ __ __	5. Occurs when muscles become fixed in one position
6.	__ __ __ I __ __	6. On the back
7.	__ __ O __ __ __ __ __	7. Steps to follow to carry out a task
8.	__ __ __ __ N __	8. Another term for orthosis

Completion

Complete the statements in the spaces provided.

1. Before beginning any patient contact, you must _____ and _____.

2. A good principle to follow is never to attempt to move a patient who weighs more than you do if you are _____.

3. A heavy or helpless patient can be more easily positioned in bed if a _____ is used.

4. A good way to help a patient maintain a side-lying position is to form a pillow roll and place it _____ _____ _____.

5. Before rolling a patient away from you, be sure the _____ _____

6. When moving the patient to the head of the bed, the nursing assistant should _____ the head of the bed.

7. The patient's position must be changed at least every _____

8. When a patient is in the prone position, the bed is in the _____ position and the patient is placed on his _____.

9. Two forms of restraint are _____ and _____.

10. When restraints are released, the patient must be _____.

11. Three incidents that may occur are _____, _____, and _____ injury.

True/False

Mark the following true or false by circling T or F.

1. T F Restraints should be used only as a last resort.

2. T F Side rails may safely be left down when restraints are in use.

3. T F Restraints should be secured to the immovable part of the bed frame.

4. T F To prevent accidental poisoning, store a patient's personal food items in the bedside table.

5. T F When preparing bath water, always turn the hot water on last.

6. T F Using a microwave oven to reheat foods is safe and economical because food is evenly heated.

7. T F Always knock before entering a room.

8. T F Special boots or shoes may be worn in bed to maintain feet in the proper alignment.

9. T F A patient positioned on her left side should be moved to the left side of the bed.

10. T F A trochanter roll should extend from under the arm, along the trunk, to the top of the hip.

Short Answer

Briefly explain the reasoning behind each of the following statements.

1. The nursing assistant should use leg muscles and shoulder muscles to lift and not the muscles of the back. Why?

   _____

   _____

   _____

2. Proper positioning of the patient's body must be conscientiously done because:

   _____

   _____

   _____

3. The staff must take specific steps before applying restraints. What are these steps and why must they be done?

   _____

   _____

   _____

Name the Position

In the space provided on the left, name the position pictured on the right.

1. _____

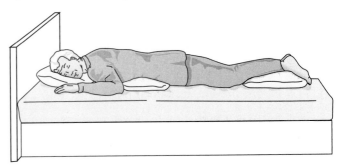

2. _____

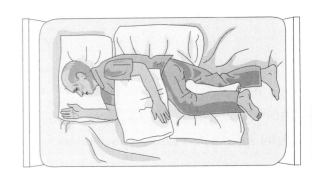

3. _____

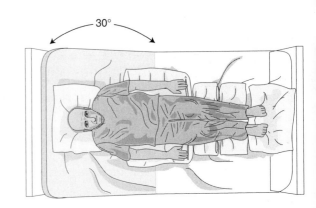

Clinical Situations

1. Mrs. Grover wears a hearing aid and glasses. She has difficulty ambulating and is unsteady on her feet. She is sometimes disoriented and tends to wander when she becomes hungry, in search of food. List ways a nursing assistant might protect this patient and avoid the need for protective restraints.

   a. _____

   b. _____

   c. _____

   d. _____

   e. _____

   f. _____

2. What might be done if physical restraint alternatives fail and the protocol for restraints has been followed?

   a. _____

   b. _____

3. Mr. Kinsey is 82 years of age, weighs 215 pounds, and has a respiratory problem (emphysema). He tends to slide to the foot of the bed and often complains of feeling uncomfortable. What action should you take when you find him in this position?

   a. _____

   b. _____

   c. _____

4. Mr. Milhouse is 91 years old and has had difficulty swallowing since his stroke. His left side is paralyzed and he needs assistance feeding himself. What might the nursing assistant do to help avoid aspiration?

   a. _____

   b. _____

   c. _____

DEVELOPING GREATER INSIGHT

1. Divide the class into groups of two or three. With one person acting as the patient, have classmates practice positioning the patient using proper supports.

2. With classmates, practice applying restraints on one another, leaving them in place for 15 minutes. Think how you would feel if you wanted a drink of water or had to use the bathroom and no one was nearby to help you.

3. With classmates, practice positioning each other in the basic patient positions.

UNIT **16**

The Patient's Mobility: Transfer Skills

OBJECTIVES

After completing this unit, you will be able to:

- Spell and define terms.
- List at least seven factors to consider, before lifting or moving a patient, to determine whether additional equipment or assistance is necessary.
- Apply the principles of good body mechanics and ergonomics to moving and transferring patients.
- List the guidelines for safe transfers.
- Describe the difference between a standing transfer and a sitting transfer.
- List the guidelines for using the manual handling sling and pivot disk.
- Demonstrate correct application and use of a transfer belt.
- Demonstrate the following procedures:

  Procedure 18 Applying a Transfer Belt

  Procedure 19 Transferring the Patient from Bed to Chair—One Assistant

  Procedure 20 Transferring the Patient from Bed to Chair—Two Assistants

  Procedure 21 Sliding-Board Transfer from Bed to Wheelchair

  Procedure 22 Transferring the Patient from Chair to Bed—One Assistant

  Procedure 23 Transferring the Patient from Chair to Bed—Two Assistants

  Procedure 24 Independent Transfer, Standby Assist

  Procedure 25 Transferring the Patient from Bed to Stretcher

  Procedure 26 Transferring the Patient from Stretcher to Bed

  Procedure 27 Transferring the Patient with a Mechanical Lift

  Procedure 28 Transferring the Patient onto and off the Toilet

UNIT SUMMARY

Assisting patients to make transfers safely is an important nursing assistant function. There are basically two types of transfers:

- Sitting transfers
- Standing transfers

The type of transfer ordered depends on the patient's:

- Strength, endurance, and balance.
- Mental condition.
- Size.

Equipment used to facilitate transfers includes:

- Transfer belts
- Mechanical lifts (hydraulic lifts), ceiling lifts, standing lifts
- Slings
- Sliders
- Sliding boards
- Swivel (pivot) disks

Transfers must be carried out smoothly, using proper body mechanics, to assure comfort and safety for both patient and worker.

NURSING ASSISTANT ALERT

Action	Benefit
Check equipment before using.	Unsafe equipment can be replaced and injury avoided.
Be sure wheelchair and bed or stretcher wheels are locked before transfer.	Prevents potential accidents, injury, and deformity.
Explain the procedure before transfer.	Enables patient to assist if possible.
Evaluate the situation and get help if needed.	Reduces patient fears. Avoids injury to patient and staff.
Use proper transfer techniques.	Avoids injury to patient and caregivers.

ACTIVITIES

Vocabulary Exercise

Complete each sentence using the best term. Select terms from the list provided.

| dependent | full weight- | gait | paralyzed |
| partial weight- | pivot | self | sitting |

1. A mechanical lift may be used to transfer a _____ patient.
2. Having the ability to stand on both legs is called _____ bearing.
3. The ability to stand on one leg is called _____ bearing.
4. A _____ patient does not have the ability to move.
5. A transfer belt is also called a _____ belt.
6. To _____ means to turn the entire body to one side.

Completion

Complete the statements in the spaces provided.

1. Before attempting to move a patient, always determine if _____ is needed.

2. Before transferring a patient from bed to chair, you should know whether the patient is _____-bearing.

3. When assisting the patient from bed to wheelchair, make sure that the footrests are _____.

4. When moving a patient with a mechanical lift, make sure the sling is positioned from _____ to _____.

5. Four people should be positioned to move an unconscious person from a stretcher to bed, as follows:

_____

_____

_____

_____

Corrections

Correct the statements that are wrong by crossing out the incorrect word or words. Write the correct words under them. Do not make any changes in the correct statements.

1. Know a patient's capabilities before attempting a transfer.

_____

2. Allow patients to place their hands around your neck.

_____

3. Use a lift sheet for standing transfers.

_____

4. Always explain the transfer plan to the patient.

_____

5. Transfer patients toward their weakest side.

_____

6. Patient shoes should have smooth soles and heels.

_____

7. Placing your hands under the patient's arms is acceptable during transfers.

_____

8. IVs, drainage bags, and other items must be considered during a transfer.

_____

9. Give patients who are transferring only the assistance they need.

_____

10. Before making a transfer, the bed should be in the high horizontal position.

_____

DEVELOPING GREATER INSIGHT

1. With classmates, practice transferring one another from bed to chair using one and then two assistants. Follow these special directions.

    a. Patient: put one arm in a sling and do not use it in the transfer.

    b. Patient: stand on right foot but bear no weight on the left.

2. Apply a transfer belt that is:

    a. too loose.

    b. too tight.

3. Practice using a mechanical lift. Select a student to act as the patient.

4. Discuss why, when assisting a patient to get up or down, the patient should not place his or her hands on the body of the nursing assistant.

The Patient's Mobility: Ambulation

OBJECTIVES

After completing this unit, you will be able to:

- Spell and define terms.
- Describe the purpose of assistive devices used in ambulation.
- List safety measures for using assistive ambulation devices.
- Describe safety measures for using a wheelchair.
- Describe nursing assistant actions for:
  - Ambulating a patient using a gait belt.
  - Propelling a patient in a wheelchair.
  - Positioning a patient in a wheelchair.
  - Transporting a patient on a stretcher.
- Demonstrate the following procedures:

  Procedure 29   Assisting the Patient to Walk with a Cane and Three-Point Gait

  Procedure 30   Assisting the Patient to Walk with a Walker and Three-Point Gait

  Procedure 31   Assisting the Falling Patient

UNIT SUMMARY

Nursing assistants frequently assist patients with ambulation. Ambulating with assistance may require the use of an assistive device. Such assistive devices include:

- Gait belt
- Walkers
- Canes
- Merry Walker
- Merry Motivator
- Merry Stand by Me (to prepare for ambulation)

Nursing assistants must be competent in applying and using assistive devices safely.

Patients also will be transported in wheelchairs, and correct techniques must be used for wheelchair use.

Nursing assistants need to follow the appropriate procedure if a patient falls.

NURSING ASSISTANT ALERT

Action	Benefit
Apply assistive devices carefully and correctly.	Contributes to patient's stability.
Use proper body mechanics when assisting a patient.	Avoids injury to patient and nursing assistant.
Learn the proper technique of two- and three-point gaits.	Provides knowledgeable support to patients who use canes and walkers.
Know and practice proper care and use of wheelchairs.	Avoids accidents and injury to patients.

ACTIVITIES

Vocabulary Exercise

Write the words that form the circle on the left and their definitions on the right.

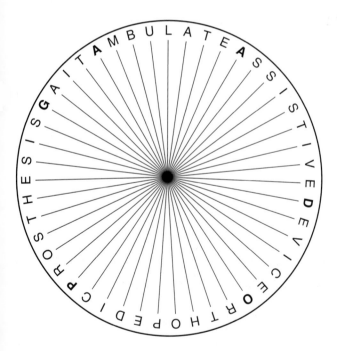

Word	Definition
1. _____	_____
2. _____	_____
3. _____	_____
4. _____	_____
5. _____	_____

Completion

Complete the following statements in the spaces provided. Select terms from the list provided.

affected	ambulation	arms	ball	four	heel
joint	need	ninety	rails	right	shoes
spills	strong	swinging	unsafe		

1. Walking is also known as _____.

2. In normal walking, the _____ strikes the floor before the _____ of the foot.

3. During walking, the arms normally have a slight _____ movement.

4. To walk safely, the patient must have adequate _____ motion.

5. The type of assistive device selected depends upon a particular patient's _____.

6. Patients should be encouraged to use hand _____ when walking.

7. When walking with a patient, the nursing assistant should stand on the patient's _____ side.

8. The nursing assistant should always check floors for clutter or _____.

9. No assistive device should be used if it is _____.

10. When forearm crutches with platforms are used, the elbows are constantly at a _____-degree angle to the shoulder.

11. When patients ambulate, clothes should not hang down over the _____.

12. A patient needs strength in both _____ to safely use a walker.

13. When ambulating with a walker, the patient shifts weight to the _____ leg as the walker is lifted and moved forward.

14. A wheelchair that fits properly will have about _____ inches between the top of the back and the patient's axillae.

15. When the feet are on the footrests of a wheelchair, the feet should be at _____ -degrees to the legs.

True/False

Mark the following true or false by circling T or F.

1. T F The arthritic patient has involuntary movements that disturb balance.
2. T F Protheses are used by patients who have had amputations, to aid mobility.
3. T F Before initiating an ambulation program, a physical therapist evaluates the patient.
4. T F If a patient requires assistance but is using a cane, a gait belt need not be used.
5. T F Quad canes provide a narrow base of support.
6. T F Canes are recommended for aiding balance rather than providing support.
7. T F A walker should be narrow so the patient can walk behind it.
8. T F The walker can safely be used as a transfer device.

9. T   F   Patients who are ambulating with a walker may use a two-point or three-point gait.

10. T   F   A wheelchair that fits the patient properly will have a two- to three-inch clearance between the front edge of the seat and the back of the patient's knees.

Short Answer

Briefly answer the statements in the spaces provided.

1. List six disorders that may affect a person's gait.

    a. _____

    b. _____

    c. _____

    d. _____

    e. _____

    f. _____

2. Identify abilities that must be evaluated by a therapist before an ambulation program may be started.

    a. _____

    b. _____

    c. _____

    d. _____

    e. _____

    f. _____

    g. _____

3. Name three commonly used assistive devices.

    a. _____

    b. _____

    c. _____

4. Explain why standard crutches are seldom recommended for older adults.

    _____

    _____

5. Explain the value of encouraging patients to do wheelchair push-ups.

    _____

6. List six guidelines for safely transporting a patient on a stretcher.

    a. _____

    b. _____

    c. _____

d. _____

e. _____

f. _____

7. List six observations to make and report about the patient's ability to ambulate and amount of assistance required.

a. _____

b. _____

c. _____

d. _____

e. _____

f. _____

Clinical Situations

Briefly describe how a nursing assistant should react to the following situations.

1. Mrs. Keane is post-stroke and weak on her left side. She uses a walker when walking. You note that the hand grip is cracked and one of the bolt nuts is missing.

_____

_____

_____

2. Mr. Jacks is using a walker for stability because he is still weak following abdominal surgery for colon cancer. You notice that he seems fatigued after walking the length of the corridor away from his room.

_____

_____

_____

3. Mrs. De Koniger is ambulating with her walker. As she moves across the room, she moves her walker 15 inches in front of her, putting her weight on her weak leg as she brings her strong foot forward.

_____

_____

_____

4. You enter Ebony Norman's room and find her on the floor. She is bleeding from somewhere on her scalp and is more confused than usual. She points at the corner and says, "He pushed me." There is no one else in the room.

_____

_____

_____

Identification

1. Circle the letter of the figure below that shows the proper way to approach a closed door with a wheelchair.

A.

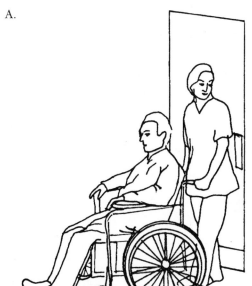

B.

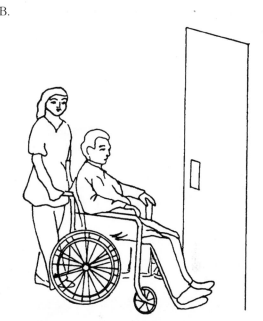

RELATING TO THE NURSING PROCESS

Write the step of the nursing process that is related to the nursing assistant action.

Nursing Assistant Action	Nursing Process Step
1. Two nursing assistants use a small sheet under the patient's buttocks to move the patient up in his wheelchair.	_____
2. The nursing assistant reports to the nurse that the patient wishes to ambulate but has only poorly fitting slippers at the bedside.	_____
3. The nursing assistant uses alcohol and cotton swabs to clean debris out of the ridges of a cane tip.	_____
4. The nursing assistant picks up old newspapers from the floor and disposes of them.	_____

DEVELOPING GREATER INSIGHT

1. Try sitting in a wheelchair for one hour without moving anything other than your arms. Discuss your reaction and concerns with your classmates.

2. Gather different types of assistive devices. Practice using them yourself. Discuss any problems with your instructor.

3. Select one student to be the patient and others to be nursing assistants. Practice assisting the "patient" who has slipped down in the wheelchair to regain proper alignment.

Measuring and Recording Vital Signs, Height, and Weight

UNIT **18**

Body Temperature

OBJECTIVES

After completing this unit, you will be able to:

- Spell and define terms.
- Identify, name, and tell the uses of the three types of clinical thermometers.
- Read a thermometer.
- Identify the range of normal temperature values.
- Demonstrate the following procedures:

  Procedure 32 Measuring an Oral Temperature (Electronic Thermometer)

  Procedure 33 Measuring a Rectal Temperature (Electronic Thermometer)

  Procedure 34 Measuring an Axillary Temperature (Electronic Thermometer)

  Procedure 35 Measuring a Tympanic Temperature

  Procedure 36 Measuring a Temporal Artery Temperature

UNIT SUMMARY

- Temperature is the measurement of body heat. It varies in different areas in the same person.

  ○ Average oral temperature is 98.6°F.

  ○ Average rectal temperature is 99.6°F.

  ○ Average axillary temperature is 97.6°F.

- Measurements of temperature may be made using the Fahrenheit (F) or Celsius (centigrade) (C) scale.

- Three kinds of clinical thermometers are commonly used to measure body temperature:
  - Oral
  - Security
  - Rectal
- There are different-colored thermometer tips for rectal and oral use.
- In addition to glass thermometers, there are other types of thermometers:
  - Battery-operated electronic thermometer. It has different-colored tips for rectal and oral use.
  - Plastic thermometer. A disposable thermometer that has dots which change color according to the body temperature. Used only for obtaining oral values.
  - Tympanic thermometer. "Ear" thermometer that has a probe which is placed in the external auditory canal to measure body temperature at the tympanic membrane.
  - Digital thermometer. Battery-operated thermometer with a probe that is placed into the patient's mouth or rectum. The reading is shown as a digital display.
  - Temporal artery thermometer. A battery-operated thermometer that measures temperature of the skin surface over the temporal artery on the forehead. Can measure temperatures from 60°F to 107.5°F.
- Follow the procedure for measuring body temperature carefully, including initial procedure actions and ending procedure actions.

NURSING ASSISTANT ALERT

Action	Benefit
Identify temperature values expressed in Fahrenheit scale.	Avoids error in measuring and recording temperature.
Be familiar with norms of temperature in different parts of the body.	Proper nursing actions can be taken when abnormal values are identified.
Hold glass and rectal, digital, tympanic, and axillary thermometers and probes in place.	Ensures accurate temperature measurement and avoids patient injury.
Be sure thermometers or probes are intact before insertion.	Prevents injury to the patient.
Record and report results accurately.	Ensures proper communication and evaluation of patient condition.

ACTIVITIES

Vocabulary Exercise

Define the words in the spaces provided.

1. body core

_____

2. body shell

_____

3. probe

_____

4. tympanic

_____

5. vital signs

_____

Completion

Complete the statements in the spaces provided.

1. The measurement of body heat is called _____.

2. Measurement of body heat is one of the vital signs. Name three others.

   a. _____

   b. _____

   c. _____

3. List eight factors that can influence body temperature.

   a. _____

   b. _____

   c. _____

   d. _____

   e. _____

   f. _____

   g. _____

   h. _____

4. In healthy adults, what is the usual daily variation in temperature?

   _____

5. When compared to adult body temperature, the temperature of children is _____ stable.

6. When using an electronic thermometer, the _____ is inserted into the patient.

7. How is the part named in the previous question protected?

   _____

8. What happens to the protector after use? _____

   _____

9. Glass thermometers are long cylindrical tubes that contain a column of _____.

10. Write the names of the two scales used to measure a temperature.

    a. _____

    b. _____

11. You enter Odelia Michaud's room to take vital signs and learn that she just returned from outside, where she was drinking gourmet coffee, eating doughnuts, and smoking with her friends. What action should you take?

_____

12. List three advantages of the tympanic thermometer.

   a. _____

   b. _____

   c. _____

13. Indicate which method of temperature determination (oral or rectal) is best in each of the following circumstances if only glass thermometers are available.

                                                                    Method

   a. Patient has diarrhea   _____

   b. Patient is confused   _____

   c. Patient cannot breathe through his nose   _____

   d. Patient has rectal bleeding   _____

   e. Patient is comatose   _____

   f. Patient has hemorrhoids   _____

   g. Patient is restless   _____

   h. Patient is a child   _____

   i. Patient has fecal impaction   _____

   j. Patient is coughing   _____

14. Name three areas other than the mouth or rectum that can be used to determine body temperature.

   a. _____

   b. _____

   c. _____

15. Write the names of the thermometers pictured.

   a. _____

b. _____

c. _____

d. _____

e. _____

True/False

Mark the following true or false by circling T or F.

1. T F   The body temperature is lower the closer to the body surface it is measured.

2. T F   The tympanic thermometer is the most accurate.

3. T F   The same person may have different temperatures when the value is determined at different parts of the body.

4. T F   Hydration levels have no effect on body temperature.

5. T F   Body heat is managed by special cells in the liver.

6. T F   The tip of a rectal thermometer should always be lubricated before insertion.

7. T F   Oxygen use will alter the temperature value of a temporal artery thermometer.

8. T F   A new disposable cover should be used to protect the electronic thermometer for each patient.

9. T F   The probe of the tympanic thermometer should be placed directly under the patient's tongue.

10. T F   A patient's temperature should be recorded as soon as it is taken.

11. T F   When taking a tympanic temperature on an adult, gently pull the ear pinna back and up.

12. T F   There is no need to cover the tip of the tympanic thermometer if you wipe it with alcohol before each use.

13. T F   Always wear gloves when taking a temporal artery temperature.

14. T F   The temporal artery thermometer measures centigrade values only.

Clinical Situations

1. Mrs. Morgan's oral temp was 98.4°F at 9:00 AM. When you see her at 10:30 AM, she is flushed and her skin is dry. What action should you take? _____

_____

2. You are assigned to recheck the temperatures of two patients using the electronic thermometer. The probe cover package is empty. You only have two temperatures to take and new covers are at the far end of the hall. What do you do? _____

_____

_____

RELATING TO THE NURSING PROCESS

Write the step of the nursing process that is related to the nursing assistant action.

Nursing Assistant Action	Nursing Process Step
1. The nursing assistant covers the digital thermometer with a disposable sheath before placing it under the patient's tongue.	_____
2. The nursing assistant accurately reports that the patient's temperature is 102°F orally.	_____

3. Before inserting a rectal thermometer, the nursing assistant lubricates the tip with water-soluble lubricant.   _____

4. The nursing assistant checks the nursing care plan before measuring an oral temperature when she notices that the patient is receiving oxygen by face mask.   _____

5. The nursing assistant reports that the patient feels faint and has hot, flushed skin.   _____

DEVELOPING GREATER INSIGHT

1. Practice taking temperatures using different types of thermometers.

2. Discuss with your instructor and classmates why proper placement of the tympanic thermometer is important.

3. Think about the times and reasons for using disposable gloves for temperature-taking procedures.

4. Explain to classmates why the forehead is a useful site for taking the temperature and explain why this value is accurate even though the temperature value is obtained on the outside of the body.

Pulse and Respiration

OBJECTIVES

After completing this unit, you will be able to:

- Spell and define terms.
- Define pulse.
- Explain the importance of monitoring a pulse rate.
- Locate the pulse sites.
- Identify the range of normal pulse and respiratory rates.
- Measure the pulse at different locations.
- List the characteristics of the pulse and respiration.
- List eight guidelines for using the stethoscope.
- Demonstrate the following procedures:

    Procedure 37   Counting the Radial Pulse

    Procedure 38   Counting the Apical-Radial Pulse

    Procedure 39   Counting Respirations

UNIT SUMMARY

- Pulse and respiration rates and character are part of the vital signs.
- The values are usually determined in a single procedure.
- Differences in apical and radial pulse rates are known as *pulse deficits*.
- Accurate values for respirations are best obtained when the patient is unaware that the procedure is being carried out.
- Unusual findings should be reported to the nurse.

NURSING ASSISTANT ALERT

Action	Benefit
Measure and record the character of pulse and respiration.	Provides important information regarding patient condition.
Recognize factors that alter pulse or respiratory rate.	Factors must be considered when evaluating findings.
Identify the norms for pulse and respiratory rates.	Proper nursing assistant actions may be taken when abnormal findings are identified.
Record findings accurately.	Ensures proper communication and evaluation of patient condition to other health care providers.

ACTIVITIES

Vocabulary Exercise

Each line has four different spellings of a word. Circle the correctly spelled word.

1.	appical	apical	apecal	apicale
2.	cyanosis	sianosis	syanosis	cyanoses
3.	poulse	pullse	polse	pulse
4.	despnea	dypnea	disnea	dyspnea
5.	apnea	epnea	apnia	appnea
6.	tachipnea	tachypnea	takipnea	tachipnia
7.	rhythm	rhythem	rhethem	rytham
8.	bradekardia	bradicardea	bradycardia	bradykardya

Completion

Complete the following statements in the spaces provided.

1. The pulse is the _____ of blood felt against the wall of an _____.

2. The pulse can be felt best in _____ that come close to the _____ and can be gently pressed against a _____.

3. You should measure the _____ pulse when the patient is unconscious.

4. Pulse measurement includes determining the pulse character, which means the _____ and _____.

5. To check circulation to the toes of your patient with diabetes, you should palpate the _____ artery.

6. Seven major arteries used to measure pulse rates are:

   a. _____

   b. _____

c. _____

d. _____

e. _____

f. _____

g. _____

7. In an adult, the normal pulse rate is between _____ bpm and _____ bpm.

8. Ten factors that can alter the pulse rate are:

   a. _____

   b. _____

   c. _____

   d. _____

   e. _____

   f. _____

   g. _____

   h. _____

   i. _____

   j. _____

9. Your patient is 8 years old and has a pulse rate of 120. You know this is _____ for a child of this age.

10. To accurately measure a pulse rate, your watch must have a _____.

11. You should locate the pulse with your _____.

12. The pulse should be counted for _____.

True/False

Mark the following true or false by circling T or F.

1. T F Normally the apical pulse is 4 bpm higher than the radial pulse in the same person.

2. T F Three health care providers are needed to accurately measure an apical pulse.

3. T F When determining an apical pulse, you will need a stethoscope.

4. T F The earpieces of the stethoscope must be cleaned before use.

5. T F Moist respirations are best documented as stertorous.

6. T F Each respiration consists of one inspiration and one expiration.

7. T F *Symmetry* of respirations refers to the depth of respiration.

8. T F The regularity of respirations is referred to as the *rhythm*.

9. T F The normal adult rate is 25 respirations per minute.

10. T F Always count the respiratory rate after you tell the patient what you intend to do.

Clinical Situations

Briefly describe how a nursing assistant should react to the following situations.

1. You are measuring vital signs and notice that the patient in 112B, whose pulse rate has been 84 to 88 bpm, now has a pulse rate of 112 and the pulse is weak.

   _____

2. Mr. Murray has a medical diagnosis of congestive heart failure. When you measure his pulse, you find it irregular and weak. The nurse says she suspects a pulse deficit.

   _____

3. You report that Mr. Rossi has a pulse deficit of 24 and a pulse rate of 84. What was the patient's apical pulse, and how would you document the reading? Show your work.

   _____

   _____

   _____

4. Find the pulse deficit in each of the following readings and show proper documentation.

   a. apical pulse 120, radial pulse 104 _____

   b. apical pulse 118, radial pulse 88 _____

   c. apical pulse 92, radial pulse 50 _____

   d. apical pulse 102, radial pulse 68 _____

   e. apical pulse 98, radial pulse 76 _____

Label the diagrams.

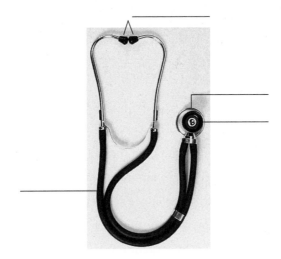

5. This piece of medical equipment is a _____.

6. Each dot on this diagram represents the location of a _____.

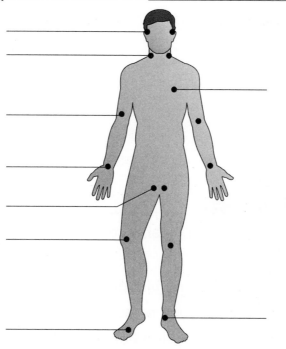

RELATING TO THE NURSING PROCESS

Write the step of the nursing process that is related to the nursing assistant action.

Nursing Assistant Action   **Nursing Process Step**

1. The nursing assistant tells the nurse that the patient's
   respirations have become labored.   _____

2. The nursing assistant has an order to measure the apical
   pulse. She seeks help because she is not sure how to
   perform this procedure.   _____

3. The nursing assistant notifies the nurse that the patient's pulse
   rate is 60.   _____

4. The nursing assistant listens closely as the nurse explains
   the new, revised care plans for her patients.   _____

5. The nursing assistant listens and counts the respirations for
   a full minute when the patient's respirations are irregular.   _____

DEVELOPING GREATER INSIGHT

1. Practice taking pulse and respiration readings on your classmates. Have your instructor check your findings.

2. Discuss ways of handling the following situations with the class:

   a. Mr. Volaire has an irregular pulse.

   b. Mrs. Benton has an IV on the thumb side of one wrist.

   c. Mrs. Zeldane seems to stop breathing shortly after you start counting the pulse, making it impossible
      for you to count her respirations.

   d. Mr. Capione's pulse and respiratory rates have increased markedly since your last measurement.

Blood Pressure

OBJECTIVES

After completing this unit, you will be able to:

- Spell and define terms.
- Describe the factors that influence blood pressure.
- Identify the range of normal blood pressure values.
- Identify the causes of inaccurate blood pressure readings.
- Select the proper size blood pressure cuff.
- List precautions associated with use of the sphygmomanometer.
- Demonstrate the following procedures:

  Procedure 40   Taking Blood Pressure

  Procedure 41   Taking Blood Pressure with an Electronic Blood Pressure
  Apparatus

UNIT SUMMARY

Blood pressure must be determined and recorded accurately by watching the gauge of the sphygmomanometer and listening with the stethoscope.

- Note and record the first regular sound as the systolic pressure.
- Note and record the change in sound or the last sound as the diastolic pressure, as directed by facility policy.

- Recheck unusual readings after one minute.
- Report unusual blood pressure to the nurse.
- Document the blood pressure as an improper fraction with the systolic reading above the diastolic reading.

NURSING ASSISTANT ALERT

Action	Benefit
Use a blood pressure cuff of proper size.	Correct readings can be obtained only if the proper size cuff is used.
Clean stethoscope earpieces before and after use.	Prevents transmission of infection between caregivers.
Do not take blood pressure on an arm that has an IV or is paralyzed.	Prevents injury to the patient.
Read the gauge at eye level.	Gives accurate reading.

ACTIVITIES

Vocabulary Exercise

Complete the puzzle by filling in the missing letters of words found in this unit. Use the definitions to help you discover these words.

1.   H
2.   _ Y _ _ _ _ _ _ _ _ _
3.   _ _ P _ _ _ _ _ _ _ _
4.   _ _ _ _ _ _ E _
5.   _ R _ _ _ _ _ _

6.   _ _ _ _ T _ _ _ _ _
7.   _ _ E _ _ _ _
8. _ _ _ _ _ _ _ _ N _ _ _ _ _ _
9.   _ _ S _ _ _ _
10.   _ _ _ _ _ _ I _
11. _ _ _ _ _ _ _ _ O _ _
12.   _ _ _ _ _ _ _ N_ _

1. unit of measurement of blood pressure
2. low blood pressure
3. drugs that slow down body function
4. felt
5. artery most often used to determine blood pressure
6. stretchability
7. type of gauge
8. blood pressure cuff and gauge
9. not eating
10. lowest blood pressure reading
11. an instrument used to hear body sounds
12. drugs that speed up body functions

Completion

Complete the statements in the spaces provided.

1. Blood pressure depends on four factors. They are:

   a. _____
   b. _____
   c. _____
   d. _____

2. List five factors other than heredity that can cause elevated blood pressure.

   a. _____
   b. _____
   c. _____
   d. _____
   e. _____

3. List five factors that can lower blood pressure, other than grief.

   a. _____

   b. _____

   c. _____

   d. _____

   e. _____

4. A properly sized blood pressure cuff should measure approximately _____ of the patient's arm.

5. Three types of sphygmomanometers in common use are:

   a. _____

   b. _____

   c. _____

6. The patient has a blood pressure reading of 148/98. You recognize this as _____.

7. The difference between the systolic and diastolic pressure is called the _____.

8. Three reasons for not using an arm to measure blood pressure are: the arm is _____, the arm is the site of an _____, or the arm is _____.

9. Sound that fades out for 10 to 15 mm Hg and then resumes as you deflate the cuff is known as

   _____.

10. The large lines on the blood pressure gauge are at increments of _____ Hg.

11. Each small line on the blood pressure gauge indicates _____ intervals.

12. The cuff should be applied _____ above the elbow.

13. The center of the rubber bladder should be placed directly over the _____.

14. Three situations that you should immediately report regarding blood pressure measurement are:

   a. _____

   b. _____

   c. _____

15. Unusual blood pressure readings ought to be checked after _____.

16. Identify the equipment and the specific parts.

   a. _____

   b. _____

   c. _____

   d. _____

   e. This is a _____

17. Determine the systolic and diastolic readings.

Systolic

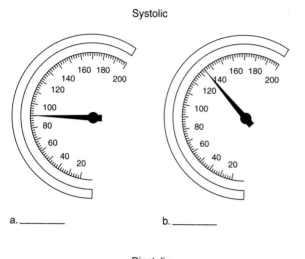

a. _____   b. _____

Diastolic

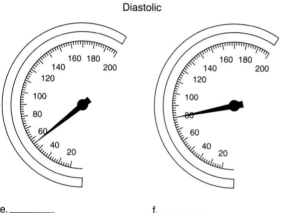

e. _____   f. _____

Systolic

c. _____

d. _____

Diastolic

g. _____

h. _____

True/False

Mark the following true or false by circling T or F.

1. T F The same size blood pressure cuff may be used for all patients.

2. T F The highest point of blood pressure measurement is the diastolic reading.

3. T F Hereditary factors can cause elevated blood pressure.

4. T F Deflating the cuff too slowly can result in an inaccurate reading.

5. T F All blood pressure readings should be made with the gauge above eye level.

6. T F The diastolic pressure is measured at the change sound or last sound that is heard.

7. T F The blood pressure is most often taken over the brachial artery.

8. T F Always clean the stethoscope earpieces and diaphragm before and after use.

9. T F Grief lowers the blood pressure.

10. T F Blood pressure readings are always recorded as a proper fraction such as 40/110.

11. T F It is very important to use a cuff of the proper size when determining the blood pressure.

12. T F A blood pressure may be measured using an arm in which an IV is inserted.

RELATING TO THE NURSING PROCESS

Write the step of the nursing process that is related to the nursing assistant action.

Nursing Assistant Action	Nursing Process Step
1. The nursing assistant finds that the patient's blood pressure is higher than the previous reading and reports this information.	_____
2. The patient is very heavy and the nursing assistant seeks guidance as to which size blood pressure cuff to use.	_____
3. The nursing assistant informs the team leader of the patient's vital signs before leaving for a break.	_____

DEVELOPING GREATER INSIGHT

1. What action is taking place in the heart when you see the systolic reading?

2. Practice taking blood pressure on patients whose arms are different sizes.

3. Explain why narrowing of the blood vessels raises blood pressure.

4. Explain why a blood pressure cuff should not be placed on the same side as a recent mastectomy.

Measuring Height and Weight

OBJECTIVES

After completing this unit, you will be able to:

- Spell and define terms.
- Understand why accurate weight measurements are important.
- Describe the proper use of an overbed scale.
- Demonstrate the following procedures:

  Procedure 42 Weighing and Measuring the Patient Using an Upright Scale

  Procedure 43 Weighing the Patient on a Chair Scale

  Procedure 44 Measuring Weight with an Electronic Wheelchair Scale

  Procedure 45 Measuring and Weighing the Patient in Bed

UNIT SUMMARY

Measurements of the patient's height and weight are usually taken on admission.

- Medications are often given according to the patient's weight.
- Weight changes may reflect the patient's condition and progress.

Measurements of height are made in:

- Feet (′)
- Inches (″)
- Centimeters (cm)

Measurements of weight are made in:

- Pounds (lb)
- Kilograms (kg)

Different techniques and equipment are used to make height and weight determinations depending on the patient's condition.

NURSING ASSISTANT ALERT

Action	Benefit
Recognize that weight may be recorded in pounds or kilograms.	Avoid errors in measuring and documenting weights
Remember that height can be measured in feet and inches or in centimeters.	Ensures correct interpretation of findings.
Always balance the scale before using.	Ensures correct weight.

ACTIVITIES

```
s   i   m   p   t   h   g   i   e   h   s
u   t   n   d   w   l   a   v   v   c   d
s   z   n   c   d   q   a   m   a   e   o
m   m   z   e   h   c   q   l   t   g   a
a   s   a   t   m   u   e   a   y   j   f
r   d   b   k   r   e   r   n   e   n   u
g   n   j   j   a   b   r   r   s   h   o
o   u   j   r   i   g   o   c   h   u   n
l   o   m   l   p   l   a   v   n   y   e
i   p   a   b   p   e   f   g   r   i   z
k   c   e   v   e   c   n   a   l   a   b
```

Completion

Complete the statements in the spaces provided. Select terms from the list provided.

bed   chair   clothing   empty   kilograms
metric   paper towel   same   scale
sling   tape measure   upright   wheelchair

1. Choose the correct scale for each patient.

   a. Mr. Graham is in a wheelchair and cannot stand. He should be weighed with a/an _____ scale.

   b. Mrs. Almos is recovering from pneumonia and is up and about as desired. She should be weighed with a/an _____ scale.

   c. Mrs. DerHagopian is elderly. Her condition requires constant bed rest. She should be weighed with a/an _____ scale.

2. Patients should be weighed at the _____ time each day.

3. Patients should wear the same type of _____ each time they are weighed.

4. The same method and _____ should be used each time a patient is weighed.

5. Patients should _____ their bladders before weighing.

6. When a patient cannot get out of bed, height measurement may be made with a _____.

7. Before weighing a patient, the platform of an upright scale should be covered with a _____.

8. Some facilities use the _____ system, which records weights in _____.

Reading Weights and Heights

Read each weight measurement and record it in pounds.

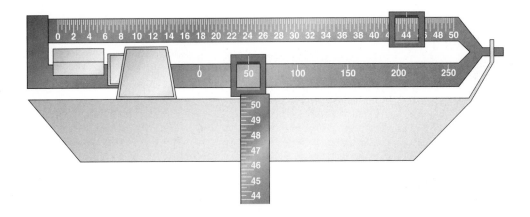

1. _____

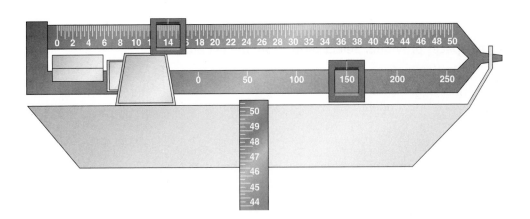

2. _____

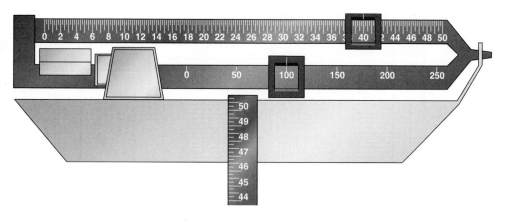

3. _____

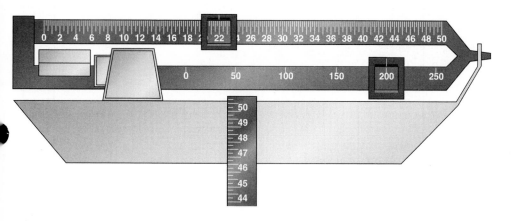

4. _____

Read each height measurement and record it in feet and inches.

1. _____

| 67 |
| 66 |
| 65 |
| 64 |
| 63 |
| 62 |
→ | 61 |
| 60 |
| 59 |
| 58 |
| 57 |
| 56 |
| 55 |

2. _____

→ | 67 |
| 66 |
| 65 |
| 64 |
| 63 |
| 62 |
| 61 |
| 60 |
| 59 |
| 58 |
| 57 |
| 56 |
| 55 |

3. _____

| 67 |
| 66 |
| 65 |
| 64 |
| 63 |
| 62 |
| 61 |
→ | 60 |
| 59 |
| 58 |
| 57 |
| 56 |
| 55 |

4. _____

| 67 |
| 66 |
| 65 |
→ | 64 |
| 63 |
| 62 |
| 61 |
| 60 |
| 59 |
| 58 |
| 57 |
| 56 |
| 55 |

True/False

Mark the following true or false by circling T or F.

1. T   F   Weights should be moved to the extreme left before weighing.

2. T   F   Patients may hold the bar while being weighed as long as they do not lean on the scale.

3. T   F   Before weighing a patient on a wheelchair scale, be sure to weigh the wheelchair only.

4. T   F   The wheels of a wheelchair need not be locked when weighing the patient on a wheelchair scale.

5. T   F   When using a bed scale, the patient's body must be suspended freely above the bed before a reading is taken.

RELATING TO THE NURSING PROCESS

Write the step of the nursing process that is related to the nursing assistant action.

Nursing Assistant Action   **Nursing Process Step**

1. The nursing assistant measures and weighs the new patient
    as instructed.   _____

2. The nursing assistant reports information about the patient's height
    and weight to the nurse and records it on the patient's record.   _____

DEVELOPING GREATER INSIGHT

1. With classmates, practice the safe use of different types of scales.

2. Explain why a patient whose height is 64 inches is recorded as 5 feet 4 inches.

3. Mrs. Menitt is a new admission. She cannot get out of bed. Think through the steps you will take to obtain an accurate height measurement.

Patient Care and Comfort Measures

U N I T **22**

Admission, Transfer, and Discharge

OBJECTIVES

After completing this unit, you will be able to:

- Spell and define terms.
- List the ways the nursing assistant can help in the processes of admission, transfer, and discharge.
- Describe family dynamics and emotions that occur when a loved one is admitted to the hospital.
- List ways in which the nursing assistant can develop positive relationships with a patient's family members.
- Demonstrate the following procedures:

  Procedure 46 Admitting the Patient

  Procedure 47 Transferring the Patient

  Procedure 48 Discharging the Patient

UNIT SUMMARY

The nursing assistant has specific responsibilities related to the admission, transfer, and discharge of the patient. These responsibilities include:

- Providing emotional support to both patient and family.

- Assisting in the safe physical transport of the patient.

- Carrying out the specific procedures related to admission, transfer, and discharge.

- Preparing and disassembling the patient unit before and after use.

- Reporting and documenting observations.

NURSING ASSISTANT ALERT

Action	Benefit
Consider needs of visitors as well as those of the new patient.	Contributes to patient and family feelings of welcome and security.
Make careful observations and accurate documentation.	Provides information essential to the formulation of an appropriate nursing care plan.

ACTIVITIES

Vocabulary Exercise

Write the words forming the circle and define them. Start at the arrow.

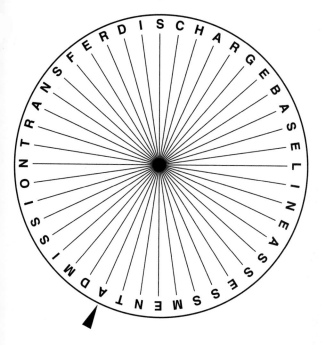

1. _____

_____

2. _____

_____

3. _____

_____

4. _____
   _____

5. _____
   _____

Completion

Complete the statements in the spaces provided.

1. Admission to a care facility is a cause of great concern for both _____ and
   _____.

2. The nursing assistant should identify the patient by speaking the patient's name and _____.

3. _____ helps identify issues that could become problematic for the patient.

4. The nursing assistant can help orient the patient to the unit by explaining how to use the telephone or television and the times _____ are served.

5. When transferring a patient to another unit, your manner should be _____ and efficient.

6. Never leave the patient, his records, or medications _____ during the transfer procedure.

7. After a transfer is completed, you should be sure the patient is _____ and
   _____.

8. Before preparing the patient for discharge, make sure the _____ has been written.

9. The nursing assistant's _____ are very valuable in the nurse's baseline assessment.

10. The patient is the facility's _____ until she has left the building.

11. After discharge, a final _____ is made on the patient chart.

12. Before the patient leaves for discharge, make sure the _____ have been given to him.

13. DRGs were introduced for the purpose of _____.

Short Answer

Briefly answer the statements in the spaces provided.

1. List six items you can expect to find in the admission kit:

   a. _____

   b. _____

   c. _____

   d. _____

   e. _____

   f. _____

2. The nursing assistant can facilitate the admission procedure if seven points are kept in mind and carried out. List them.

a. _____

b. _____

c. _____

d. _____

e. _____

f. _____

g. _____

3. Before admitting the patient, you will need specific information. What questions should you ask the nurse?

a. _____

b. _____

c. _____

Clinical Situations

Briefly describe how a nursing assistant should react to the following situations.

1. Your patient tells you he intends to leave the health care facility without his physician's permission.

_____

2. Your patient has just been discharged.

_____

_____

_____

3. The family accompanies your patient to the unit and must wait as you carry out the admission procedure. How can you show courtesy to them?

_____

_____

_____

_____

_____

4. Your assignment is to admit the patient to Room 16C. List the equipments you will gather.

_____

_____

_____

_____

_____

RELATING TO THE NURSING PROCESS

Write the step of the nursing process that is related to the nursing assistant action.

Nursing Assistant Action	Nursing Process Step
1. The nursing assistant carefully prepares the patient's unit before admission.	_____
2. The nursing assistant measures the vital signs during the admission procedure.	_____
3. During admission, the nursing assistant carefully observes the patient and listens to the patient's statements.	_____
4. The nursing assistant makes sure that all the patient's personal articles are transported to the new unit when the patient is transferred.	_____
5. The nursing assistant documents the correct time and method of patient discharge on the proper record.	_____

DEVELOPING GREATER INSIGHT

1. With classmates, role-play the following situations (consider equipment, psychological, and physical needs):

    a. Mrs. Coe is being admitted. She is in a wheelchair and very frail.

    b. Mr. Fletcher is ambulatory and is being discharged to the care of his son and daughter-in-law. The daughter-in-law seems very nervous and is pacing back and forth.

    c. Mrs. Barkley spends most of the day in a wheelchair. She is to be transferred to another floor.

Bedmaking

OBJECTIVES

After completing this unit, you will be able to:

- Spell and define terms.
- List the different types of beds and their uses.
- Operate each type of bed.
- Properly handle clean and soiled linens.
- Demonstrate the following procedures:

  Procedure 49 Making a Closed Bed

  Procedure 50 Opening the Closed Bed

  Procedure 51 Making an Occupied Bed

  Procedure 52 Making the Surgical Bed

UNIT SUMMARY

Proper bedmaking is an important part of your work.

- A skillfully made bed provides comfort and safety for the patient.
- Beds may be built to meet specific patient needs and conditions. Each type of bed will be made differently.
- Common types of beds include:
  - Low air loss
  - Electric
  - Gatch
  - Low
  - Specialty beds

- Bedmaking methods include:
  - Closed bed
  - Occupied bed
  - Unoccupied bed
  - Surgical bed
- Draw sheets (turning sheets) may be used, depending on patient requirements.
- Many facilities use fitted bottom sheets. The bedmaking procedure may be modified to accommodate this difference.

NURSING ASSISTANT ALERT

Action	Benefit
Handle linen carefully and properly.	Prevents spread of germs.
Raise bed to comfortable working height during procedure.	Reduces strain on caregiver.
Make bed neatly and smoothly.	Contributes to comfort and lessens chance of (pressure) ulcer formation.
Know how to operate bed and equipment before attempting to do so.	Avoids injury to patient and caregiver.
Always leave bed in lowest horizontal position.	Reduces the possibility of falls and accidents when patient gets in and out of bed.
Use standard precautions if contact with blood, body fluids, secretions, or excretions is likely.	Prevents spread of germs. Protects caregiver, patient, and others by reducing environmental germs.

ACTIVITIES

Vocabulary Exercise

Unscramble the words introduced in this unit and define them.

1. Y R T R E S K _____

   _____

2. H A C G T _____

   _____

3. T S O B X E P A L _____

   _____

4. I E T D R E M _____

   _____

5. F F A O N L D _____

   _____

6. I R S E A D L I S _____

   _____

7. E T H E S _____

   _____

True/False

Mark the following true or false by circling T or F.

1. T   F   Gatch beds are most commonly used in home health care.

2. T   F   After the bottom of the bed has been made, pull the mattress to the head of the bed.

3. T F   Before making a bed, lower it to its lowest horizontal height.

4. T F   When completing an open bed, position the top bedding under the pillow.

5. T F   The top linen of a surgical bed is left untucked and fanfolded to one side.

6. T F   Position the lift sheet from the patient's waist to his knees.

7. T F   CPR is not effective on a low-air-loss bed.

8. T F   The risk of side rail entrapment increases in low-air-loss beds.

9. T F   A mattress pad is applied to the mattress before the bottom sheet is put on.

10. T F   Fitted sheets are used in some facilities in place of top sheets.

11. T F   Before making an unoccupied bed, arrange the linen in the order it is to be used.

12. T F   Always position a patient comfortably before leaving the room.

13. T F   The flat bottom sheet should be placed so the bottom edge is even with the end of the mattress at the foot of the bed.

14. T F   Place the clean bed linen on the overbed table.

15. T F   Never shake the linen when making a bed, because this may spread germs.

16. T F   When making the bottom of an occupied bed, the linen should be rolled against the patient's back and then tucked under the patient's body.

17. T F   Loosen the top linen when a bed is occupied.

18. T F   Side rails should be up and secure before you leave an occupied bed.

Identification

Identify the following items.

1. Name the type of corner that has been made in the linen.

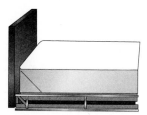

2. Identify the type of bed pictured here.

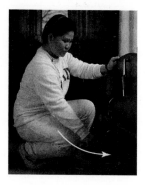

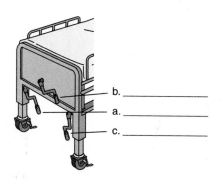

b. _____

a. _____

c. _____

State the purpose of each handle at the foot of the bed:

a. _____

b. _____

c. _____

3. Identify the items pictured here.

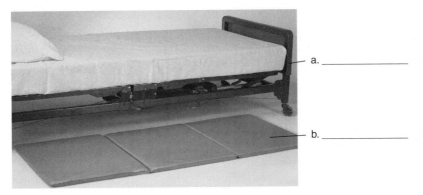

a. _____

b. _____

4. a. Name the fold the nursing assistant is making in the linen.

_____

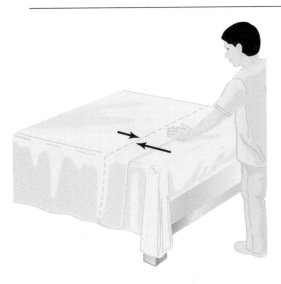

b. State the purpose of folding the linen in this manner.

_____

Short Answer

Briefly answer the following questions.

1. Why should one side of the bed be made at a time?

_____

2. Why are the sheets unfolded rather than shaken out?

_____

3. How should the pillow be placed on the bed?

_____

4. What is the purpose of the open bed?

_____

5. What is the purpose of the surgical bed?

_____

6. Why is it important to screen the patient unit before beginning to make an occupied bed?

_____

7. Why is it necessary to turn patients who are in low-air-loss beds that reduce pressure on the skin?

_____

8. What is the proper position for the overbed table when the bed is closed or unoccupied?

_____

9. When is the closed bed made in the hospital?

_____

10. Why would the wheels of the bed be locked before the nursing assistant starts to make the bed?

_____

11. Complete the following chart.

Method of Bedmaking	Procedure Variations	Rationale
Unoccupied bed	a. Most _____ type of bedmaking procedure • Used for making all types of beds	b. Making the unoccupied bed is _____ and faster for the nursing assistant. It is more comfortable for the patient.
Occupied bed	c. Used when the patient is _____ to bed.	Changes wet or soiled linen for patient comfort and prevention of skin breakdown. Provides fresh, clean linen for feeling of comfort and security.
d. _____ bed	• The bed is made with the top sheet, blanket, and spread pulled all the way to the top. • The pillow may be covered or placed on top of the spread, depending on facility policy. • The open end of the pillowcase faces away from the door.	e. Used when the patient is expected to be _____ all day or when making a bed after the patient has been discharged. Presents a neat, tidy appearance.
Open bed	• The bed is made in the normal manner. f. The top sheet and spread are _____ to the foot of the bed.	This procedure is used when the patient is temporarily out of bed. The patient or nursing assistant can easily and quickly cover the patient upon return to bed.

CLINICAL SITUATIONS

Briefly describe how a nursing assistant should react to the following situations.

1. You finish making the occupied bed and you notice that the bed is at the working horizontal height.

   _____

   _____

2. Your patient, Shon Fajardo, asks you to raise the side rails before leaving the room so she can pull on them when she moves.

   _____

   _____

3. A visitor tells you that her father is to be placed on a low-air-loss bed and asks you what kind of bed that is.

   _____

   _____

4. You finish giving Kia Florez a bath and find you have an extra clean towel that was not used. What should be done with the towel?

   _____

   _____

Answer the questions about the clinical situation. Briefly explain your answers.

It is career day for your local high school. The nurse manager of your unit has asked you to allow a high school student to "shadow" you during your shift. You know that only the best nursing assistants are asked to work with these students and you feel honored to be asked. The student, who is close to your age, is glad to be there and very excited to be working with you. She has many questions. The student asks you the following:

5. What is the purpose of the low bed in room 321?

   _____

   _____

6. What is the purpose of the mat on the floor next to the low bed?

   _____

   _____

7. Doesn't it hurt your back to care for the patient in the low bed and make the bed while bending over? What can you do to prevent a backache?

   _____

   _____

   _____

   _____

8. Why do you elevate the electric hospital bed when you are making the bed?

   _____

   _____

9. Why do you lower the bed when you have finished making it?

   _____

   _____

10. Why did you leave the room to put the soiled bed linen in the hamper in the hallway? Wouldn't it be easier to put it on the floor and take it to the hamper when you have finished?

_____

_____

_____

11. What is the purpose of the half sheet in the center of the bed?

_____

_____

12. After you finished making the bed, you pulled the top linen down and folded it at the foot of the bed. That seems like undoing what you just finished. Why did you do this?

_____

_____

_____

_____

13. Why do you make one side of a bed at a time?

_____

_____

_____

RELATING TO THE NURSING PROCESS

Write the step of the nursing process that is related to the nursing assistant action.

Nursing Assistant Action   **Nursing Process Step**

1. The nursing assistant makes sure the bottom bed linen is free of wrinkles.

    _____

2. The nursing assistant applies gloves before removing wet and soiled bed linen.

    _____

3. The nursing assistant makes sure the patient is not exposed when the bed linen is changed.

    _____

4. The nursing assistant is assigned to prepare a bed for a postoperative patient. She has not done this before and asks the nurse for clarification.

    _____

DEVELOPING GREATER INSIGHT

1. Wrinkle the bottom linen on a bed. Make sure there are wrinkles. Put on your nightwear and spend 30 minutes on the wrinkles.

2. Make the top linen very tight. Be sure to tuck in the top sheet and spread tightly. Spend 30 minutes in this bed.

3. Discuss with classmates the reasons why making beds would be very fatiguing if proper procedures were not followed.

4. Discuss with classmates the importance of turning and repositioning patients who are in low-air-loss beds.

UNIT **24**

Patient Bathing

OBJECTIVES

After completing this unit, you will be able to:

- Spell and define terms.
- Describe the safety precautions for patient bathing.
- List the purposes of bathing patients.
- State the value of whirlpool baths.
- Demonstrate the following procedures:

  Procedure 53   Assisting with the Tub Bath or Shower

  Procedure 54   Bed Bath

  Procedure 55   Changing the Patient's Gown

  Procedure 56   Waterless Bed Bath

  Procedure 57   Partial Bath

  Procedure 58   Female Perineal Care

  Procedure 59   Male Perineal Care

  Procedure 60   Hand and Fingernail Care

  Procedure 61   Bed Shampoo

  Procedure 62   Dressing and Undressing the Patient

UNIT SUMMARY

Bathing makes a patient feel refreshed and clean. Full or partial baths may be carried out in:

- Bed
- Shower
- Regular bathtub
- Whirlpool tub

Personal hygiene measures include:

- Care of the teeth
- Care of the hair
- Care of the nails
- Dressing and undressing

Encourage patients to participate in personal hygiene measures and selection of clothing. Range-of-motion exercises are frequently performed during the bath procedure, according to the patient's needs and orders. (See Unit 41.) The daily hygiene routine gives you a chance to make close observations of the patient.

NURSING ASSISTANT ALERT

Action	Benefit
Guard against falls.	Avoids potential injury.
Maintain an even room temperature.	Prevents chilling and discomfort.
Avoid unnecessary exposure.	Protects patient's dignity and privacy.
Work quickly and smoothly, using proper body mechanics.	Lessens patient and caregiver fatigue.

ACTIVITIES

Vocabulary Exercises

Each line has four different spellings of a word. Circle the correctly spelled word.

1. cutical   cuticule   cuticale   cuticle

2. axilla   axiller   axella   arxilla

3. genetala   genitalia   genetalea   ginetalia

4. middriff   medrif   midriff   midreff

5. pubic   pubec   pobic   paobic

6. Draw a line from the word in the center to the correct scrambled word on the sides.

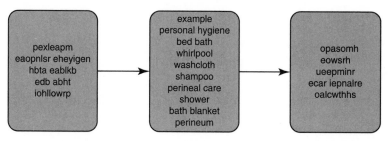

	example	
pexleapm	personal hygiene	opasomh
eaopnlsr eheyigen	bed bath	eowsrh
hbta eablkb	whirlpool	ueepminr
edb abht	washcloth	ecar iepnalre
iohllowrp	shampoo	oalcwthhs
	perineal care	
	shower	
	bath blanket	
	perineum	

Completion

Complete the statements in the spaces provided.

1. In addition to bathing the body, morning care includes cleaning the teeth, _____, and _____.

2. A partial bath ensures cleansing of the hands, face, _____, buttocks, and _____.

3. The best temperature for bath water is about _____ °F.

4. A _____ should be in the bath area in case of an emergency.

5. After the tub bath is completed and the patient has returned to the unit, return to the tub room and _____ the tub.

6. To provide privacy during a tub bath or shower, the patient may use a _____ to wrap around his _____.

7. Hold a _____ around the patient to provide privacy as he steps out of the tub.

8. Privacy can be provided during a bed bath by _____.

9. Offer the patient a _____ before giving a bath.

10. When preparing the patient for a bed bath, remove the top bedding and replace it with a _____.

11. Do not use soap near the _____.

12. Clean and wipe the eyes from _____ to _____ corner.

13. Pay special attention to the folds under a female patient's _____ as you wash her.

14. A bag bath may be used instead of using _____.

15. Apply _____ to the feet of a patient with dry skin.

16. Clip the fingernails _____ and do not clip below the _____.

17. When finishing the bath for the male patient, carefully wash and dry the _____, _____, and groin area.

18. The whirlpool tub provides the beneficial action of a _____ in addition to cleaning.

19. Allow the patient to soak the feet for _____ minutes.

20. Two abnormalities you might note during foot care are _____ and calluses.

21. When giving a bed shampoo, _____ the scalp with your _____.

22. Protect the patient's eyes with a _____ during a shampoo.

23. Dry the hair following a shampoo with a _____ or portable hair dryer.

Short Answer

Briefly answer the following questions.

1. Three values patients derive from a bath include:

    a. _____

    b. _____

    c. _____

2. Three precautions you should take when the patient is able to bathe himself in a tub include:

    a. _____

    b. _____

    c. _____

3. Special care must be given during the bath to the patient who:

   a. _____

   b. _____

   c. _____

4. There are 13 ending procedure (procedure completion) actions. They are:

   a. _____

   b. _____

   c. _____

   d. _____

   e. _____

   f. _____

   g. _____

   h. _____

   i. _____

   j. _____

   k. _____

   l. _____

   m. _____

5. List at least five situations in which gloves must be worn when bathing a patient.

   a. _____

   b. _____

   c. _____

   d. _____

   e. _____

6. Describe how a bath mitt is made.

   _____

   _____

   _____

7. List three advantages to using the waterless bathing system compared with a regular bed bath.

   a. _____

   b. _____

   c. _____

8. Why should the patient help you with the bed bath as much as his condition permits?

   _____

   _____

9. What is the nursing assistant's responsibility when the patient is unable to complete her bath?

   _____

   _____

10. What other procedures may be carried out in conjunction with the bath procedure?

    _____

11. What are four advantages of the whirlpool bath?

    a. _____

    b. _____

    c. _____

    d. _____

12. What measures can be taken to help avoid patient falls during tub bathing?

    a. _____

    b. _____

    c. _____

    d. _____

    e. _____

    f. _____

    g. _____

CLINICAL SITUATIONS

Briefly describe how a nursing assistant should react to the following situations.

1. Your patient feels weak or faint during a tub bath.

   _____

   _____

2. You have not yet finished bathing the legs of a bed patient and the water feels cool.

   _____

   _____

3. Your patient has diabetes and his toenails need cutting.

   _____

   _____

4. Describe the technique to be used when washing the penis and scrotum.

   _____

   _____

RELATING TO THE NURSING PROCESS

Write the step of the nursing process that is related to the nursing assistant action.

Nursing Assistant Action	Nursing Process Step

1. The nursing assistant carefully cleans the tub before and after each patient use.

   _____

2. The nursing assistant has to bathe a patient who has an IV line and is not sure how to remove the patient's gown. She asks a nurse for help.

   _____

3. The nursing assistant offers a bedpan to the patient before giving a bed bath.

   _____

4. The nursing assistant finds that the patient cannot separate her legs sufficiently to allow good perineal care, so the assistant asks the nurse for directions on how to give care.

   _____

5. The nursing assistant is giving foot care to a patient with thick, long toenails. He asks the nurse if the nails should be cut.

   _____

6. The nursing assistant listens carefully as the nurse explains that the care plan for a bed bath will be modified the next day to allow the patient to shower if she feels well enough.

   _____

DEVELOPING GREATER INSIGHT

1. Discuss why frequent perineal care is important to the patient's hygiene.

2. Discuss why nursing assistants are not permitted to cut the toenails of a diabetic patient.

3. Discuss ways to give perineal care if the patient cannot separate his or her legs.

4. Working with another student, demonstrate the proper way to assist a person to put on a shirt that slips over the head when the patient cannot use one side of her body.

5. Think through the reasons why you should be ready to assist patients to put on shoes and socks.

General Comfort Measures

OBJECTIVES

After completing this unit, you will be able to:

- Spell and define terms.
- Discuss the reasons for early morning and bedtime care.
- Identify patients who require frequent oral hygiene.
- List the purposes of oral hygiene.
- Explain nursing assistant responsibilities for a patient's dentures.
- State the purpose of backrubs.
- Describe safety precautions when shaving a patient.
- Describe the importance of hair care.
- Explain the use of comfort devices.
- State the purpose of bed boards and list guidelines for their use.
- Demonstrate the following procedures:

  Procedure 63   Assisting with Routine Oral Hygiene

  Procedure 64   Assisting with Special Oral Hygiene—Dependent and Unconscious Patients

  Procedure 65   Assisting the Patient to Floss and Brush Teeth

  Procedure 66   Caring for Dentures

  Procedure 67   Backrub

  Procedure 68   Shaving a Male Patient

  Procedure 69   Daily Hair Care

  Procedure 70   Giving and Receiving the Bedpan

  Procedure 71   Giving and Receiving the Urinal

  Procedure 72   Assisting with Use of the Bedside Commode

4. Why should nursing assistants keep their fingernails short?

_____

5. Why should the skin be held taut while using the razor?

_____

6. What would you do if you accidentally nicked a patient during the shaving procedure?

_____

7. What action would you take if a patient's hair was tangled?

_____

8. Why must gloves be worn when shaving a patient's intact face with a disposable razor?

_____

9. Six patients requiring special oral hygiene are those who are:

a. _____

b. _____

c. _____

d. _____

e. _____

f. _____

10. Five times when backrubs are usually given are:

a. _____

b. _____

c. _____

d. _____

e. _____

11. List the equipment you would need to give a backrub.

a. _____

b. _____

c. _____

d. _____

12. Why is mouth care given before the patient has breakfast?

_____

13. Why is a backrub given to the patient at bedtime?

_____

14. How do you wake the patient?

_____

15. Two instances when you would not waken the patient before breakfast are if she is:

a. _____

b. _____

16. Four activities you will carry out as part of bedtime care include:

   a. _____

   b. _____

   c. _____

   d. _____

Identifying Strokes

Using a colored pencil or crayon, draw in the indicated strokes.

1. Soothing

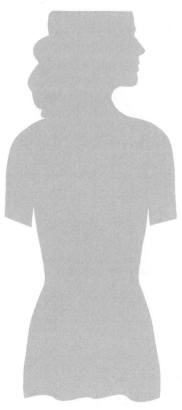

c. _____

d. _____

Clinical Situations

Briefly describe how a nursing assistant should react to the following situations.

1. You note a pressure area on your patient's hip while giving a backrub.

   _____

   _____

2. You must wash the hair of an African American patient who vomited while in bed. Some of the vomitus accidentally got in her hair. The patient has a comb, brush, and elastic hair ties, but did not bring any hair care products to the hospital. What hair care products will you need to wash, detangle, dry, and style her hair?

   _____

   _____

3. Your patient needs to use the bedpan, but cannot lift her buttocks off the bed.

   _____

   _____

4. You are giving PM care and the patient says he would like to finish the chapter he is reading.

   _____

   _____

5. Your patient is settled for the night and you are ready to leave the room.

   _____

   _____

RELATING TO THE NURSING PROCESS

Write the step of the nursing process that is related to the nursing assistant action.

Nursing Assistant Action	Nursing Process Step
1. The nursing assistant allows the patient to sleep and omits early am care because the patient is going to surgery.	_____
2. The nursing assistant makes sure that bedtime care has been given before the nurse administers sleep medications.	_____
3. The nursing assistant uses cool water when brushing the dentures for the patient.	_____
4. The nursing assistant reports that the patient's lips are very dry and cracked.	_____
5. The nursing assistant listens carefully when the patient says that he does not want to put his dentures in because they hurt.	_____
6. The nursing assistant reports and documents the condition of the patient's skin each time she gives back care.	_____

Principles of Nutrition and Fluid Balance

UNIT **26**

Nutritional Needs and Diet Modifications

OBJECTIVES

After completing this unit, you will be able to:

- Spell and define terms.
- Define normal nutrition.
- List the essential nutrients.
- Name the food groups and list the foods included in each group.
- Identify the basic facility diets and describe each.
- State the purposes of the following diets:
  - clear liquid
  - full liquid
  - soft
  - mechanically altered
- State the purpose of calorie counts and food intake studies.
- Define dysphagia and explain the risks of this condition.
- Describe general care for the patient with dysphagia and swallowing problems.
- State the purposes of therapeutic diets.

8. Four examples of incomplete proteins are:

    a. _____

    b. _____

    c. _____

    d. _____

9. Six minerals needed in any person's daily diet include:

    a. _____

    b. _____

    c. _____

    d. _____

    e. _____

    f. _____

10. Four functions of vitamins are to:

    a. _____

    b. _____

    c. _____

    d. _____

11. Six vitamins needed by the body are:

    a. _____

    b. _____

    c. _____

    d. _____

    e. _____

    f. _____

12. Name the five "P" foods to be avoided in a low-sodium diet.

    a. _____

    b. _____

    c. _____

    d. _____

    e. _____

13. What are the amounts of average servings?

    a. Fruit _____

    b. Cooked fruit or vegetable _____

    c. Meat _____

    d. Pasta/bread _____

14. A person who is receiving a consistent carbohydrate diet receives about:

    a. _____% of the daily calories from fat.

    b. _____% of the daily calories from protein.

    c. _____% of the daily calories from carbohydrate.

15. What is the purpose of serving nutritional supplements?

    _____

    _____

16. Explain the difference between supplements and nourishments.

    _____

    _____

    _____

    _____

17. Hot foods must be served at _____°F or above, and cold foods must be served at _____°F or below.

18. Explain why the food cart must be separated from the soiled linen hamper and housekeeping cart by at least one room's width in the hallways.

    _____

    _____

    _____

    _____

19. List three things you can do to maintain food temperature when the food cart arrives on the unit.

    a. _____

    b. _____

    c. _____

20. Explain the difference between a PEG tube and a nasogastric tube, and state the purpose of each tube.

    _____

    _____

21. Intake and output records are kept for six special circumstances when specifically ordered, such as in patients who:

    a. _____

    b. _____

    c. _____

    d. _____

    e. _____

    f. _____

22. Output that must be recorded includes:

    a. _____

    b. _____

a. _____

b. _____

c. _____

d. _____

e. _____

RELATING TO THE NURSING PROCESS

Write the step of the nursing process that is related to the nursing assistant action.

Nursing Assistant Action	Nursing Process Step
1. The nursing assistant carefully checks the patient's identification band against the diet slip.	_____
2. The nursing assistant reports to the nurse that the patient ate only one-third of the soft diet ordered.	_____
3. The nursing assistant documents that the patient refused lunch because he felt nauseated.	_____
4. The nursing assistant carefully records the fluids taken by the patient who has an order for I&O.	_____
5. The nursing assistant checks with the team leader to be sure gelatin should be recorded as fluid intake.	_____
6. The nursing assistant makes a special note during report that her patient is on I&O.	_____

DEVELOPING GREATER INSIGHT

1. Make a statement to the class about the actions you would take if:

   a. Your patient is on I&O and you find a container of milk one-third full when you pick up trays.

   b. Your patient is on I&O and has perspired so much during the night that you had to change the pillowcase and bottom sheet. Describe what you will monitor for the rest of your shift.

2. Try to identify the feelings you might experience if you were an Orthodox Jew and pork roast was served to you.

3. Think through what action you might take while caring for a Roman Catholic patient who is to receive Communion at 8:00 AM, when breakfast is served at 7:00 AM.

4. Working in groups, plan how you would modify the regular diet for an 82-year-old, 110-pound woman who has trouble chewing because her dentures are loose.

5. Practice feeding and being fed. Wear a clothing protector. Discuss your feelings during the experience. Consider adding a blindfold to the person being fed. Describe your experience feeding a "blind" person. Describe how it felt to be unable to see what you were eating.

6. Sample each of your facility diets (including pureed) and supplements.

Special Care Procedures

Warm and Cold Applications

OBJECTIVES

After completing this unit, you will be able to:

- Spell and define terms.
- List the physical conditions requiring the use of heat and cold.
- Name types of heat and cold applications.
- Describe the effects of local cold applications.
- Describe the effects of local heat applications.
- List safety concerns related to application of heat and cold.
- Demonstrate the following procedures:

  Procedure 76 Applying an Ice Bag or Gel Pack

  Procedure 77 Applying a Disposable Cold Pack

  Procedure 78 Applying an Aquamatic K-Pad

  Procedure 79 Giving a Sitz Bath

  Procedure 80 Assisting with Application of an Aquathermia Blanket

UNIT SUMMARY

Nursing assistants sometimes perform treatments with heat and cold. These applications must be performed cautiously, according to facility policy and the patient's care plan. Performance of warm and cold applications is a nursing assistant function only as permitted by state law.

Assisting with the Physical Examination

OBJECTIVES

After completing this unit, you will be able to:

- Spell and define terms.
- Describe the responsibilities of the nursing assistant during the physical examination.
- Name the various positions for physical examinations.
- Drape the patient for the various positions.
- Name the basic instruments necessary for physical examinations.

UNIT SUMMARY

In most facilities, two staff members must be present during a physical examination. The nursing assistant may assist the health care provider during the physical examination and as the nurse performs a nursing assessment. You do this successfully when you:

- Provide privacy while the patient's history is discussed.
- Are ready to assist during the examination and to provide proper lighting.
- Avoid overexposing the patient as you adjust the drapes.

- Remember that most patients feel uneasy about physical examinations. Be reassuring.
- Drape and position patients safely while maintaining proper body mechanics.
- Know and prepare the proper equipment for the examination.
- Assist patients during the examination and after the examination is completed.
- Properly clean up the room and equipment after the examination is completed.

NURSING ASSISTANT ALERT

Action	Benefit
Position patients for optimum comfort, safety, and privacy.	Prevents injury. Reduces anxiety. Facilitates the examination.
Have all necessary equipments and supplies ready.	Saves time. Reduces patient stress.
Stay beside and assist patients during position changes.	Provides support and prevents injury.

ACTIVITIES

Vocabulary Exercise

Each line has four different spellings of a word. Circle the correctly spelled word.

1. litotomy	lithotomy	lythotomy	lithotome
2. percussun	percussion	percusion	pacussion
3. autoscope	otascop	otoscope	otascope
4. speculum	specalum	spiculum	specolom
5. opthalomoscope	ophthalmoscope	ophtalmoscope	ophtholmascope

Definitions

Define the following words.

1. dorsal recumbent _____

2. drape _____

3. flexed _____

4. percussion hammer _____

5. ophthalmoscope _____

6. otoscope _____

7. speculum _____

Completion

Complete the following statements in the spaces provided.

1. When in the lithotomy position, the patient's knees are _____.

2. When in the dorsal recumbent position, the patient lies on his _____.

3. When in the knee-chest position, the patient should never be _____.

4. When in the prone position, the patient lies on her _____.

5. When in Sims' position, the patient lies on his _____ side.

6. The basic examination position is _____.

7. The position used for a pelvic examination is _____.

8. The position sometimes used for a rectal examination is the _____.

9. Patients are usually draped in cloth or paper _____.

10. However the draping is done, it is important that the patient _____ covered.

11. The most common position for head and neck examination is _____.

12. Name the positions pictured.

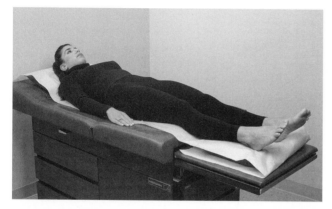

a. _____

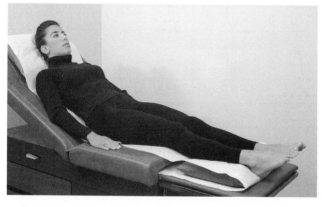

b. _____

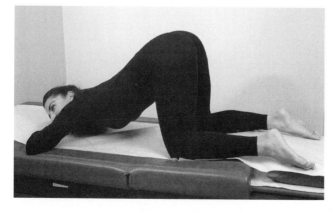

c. _____

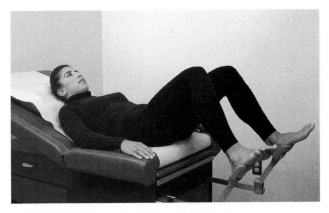

d. _____

Short Answer

Briefly explain each of the following.

1. The role of the nursing assistant during a physical examination.

_____

_____

_____

2. How the physical examination helps the physician?

_____

_____

_____

3. List the equipment you will set up for a pelvic examination.

a. _____

b. _____

c. _____

d. _____

e. _____

f. _____

g. _____

h. _____

i. _____

4. Name the instruments and equipment in a physical examination and explain the use of each.

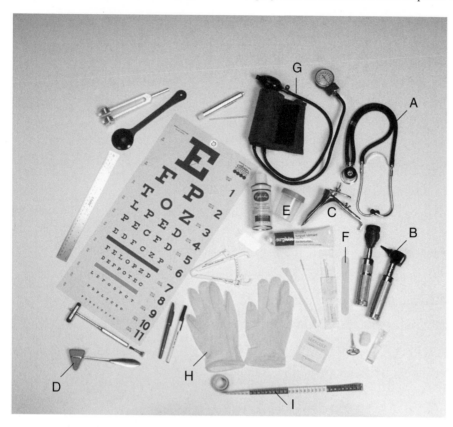

a. _____

b. _____

c. _____

d. _____

e. _____

f. _____

g. _____

h. _____

i. _____

Clinical Situations

Briefly describe how a nursing assistant should react to the following situations.

1. The patient seems very nervous before a physical examination. _____

_____

_____

2. The physician wants to do a pelvic examination. _____

_____

_____

3. The nurse wants to examine the patient's throat and chest. _____

_____

_____

True/False

Mark the following true or false by circling T or F.

1. T   F   A physical examination helps the physician establish a diagnosis.

2. T   F   The nursing assistant examines the patient to make a nursing diagnosis.

3. T   F   The nursing assistant should expose only the part being examined.

4. T   F   The nursing assistant does not need to know how to operate the examination table, because the physician will perform this task.

5. T   F   When in the horizontal recumbent position, the patient is placed on her abdomen.

6. T   F   The semi-Fowler's position is often used when the head and neck are to be examined.

7. T   F   Patients should void before the pelvic examination.

8. T   F   A Pap smear is usually taken with the patient in the semi-Fowler's position.

9. T   F   Provide privacy before the examination begins.

10. T   F   The nursing assistant should try to anticipate the examiner's needs.

RELATING TO THE NURSING PROCESS

Write the step of the nursing process that is related to the nursing assistant action.

Nursing Assistant Action	Nursing Process Step
1. The nursing assistant helps the patient assume the dorsal lithotomy position for a pelvic examination.	_____
2. The nursing assistant records information as the health care provider carries out the examination.`	_____
3. The nursing assistant measures the patient's height and weight and passes instruments during the physical examination.	_____

DEVELOPING GREATER INSIGHT

1. Try positioning yourself in the knee-chest and lithotomy positions. Think carefully of how you feel. What might be done to increase your feelings of privacy and security?

2. Ask your instructor to let you try on a hospital or examination gown. Did you feel covered?

3. Examine the instruments used for the physical examination. Describe their purposes to your classmates.

The Surgical Patient

OBJECTIVES

After completing this unit, you will be able to:

- Spell and define terms.
- Describe the concerns of patients who are about to have surgery.
- List the various types of anesthesia.
- Shave the area to be operated on.
- Prepare the patient's unit for the patient's return from the operating room.
- Give routine postoperative care when the patient returns to the room.
- Describe the care and observations for surgical drains.
- Assist the patient with deep breathing and coughing.
- Apply elasticized stockings or bandages and pneumatic hosiery.
- Demonstrate the following procedures:

  Procedure 81   Assisting the Patient to Deep Breathe and Cough

  Procedure 82   Performing Postoperative Leg Exercises

  Procedure 83   Applying Elasticized Stockings

  Procedure 84   Applying an Elastic Bandage

  Procedure 85   Applying Pneumatic Compression Hosiery

  Procedure 86   Assisting the Patient to Dangle

UNIT SUMMARY

The surgical patient requires continuous care before, during, and after surgery. The nursing assistant helps in preoperative and postoperative care.

Nursing assistant responsibilities in the preoperative period include:

- Preparing the operative site.

- Readying the patient on the morning of surgery.

- Helping transfer the patient to and from the stretcher.

- Providing emotional support.

Nursing assistant responsibilities during the operative period include:

- Preparing a surgical (postoperative) bed.
- Securing equipment needed for the postoperative period.

Nursing assistant responsibilities in the postoperative period include:

- Assisting in the transfer from stretcher to bed.
- Carefully observing and reporting.
- Monitoring vital signs frequently, as directed by the nurse or according to facility policy.

- Assisting the patient with postoperative exercises, including:
  - Position changes.
  - Leg exercises.
  - Respiratory exercises.
- Applying elasticized stockings.
- Assisting in dangling and initial ambulation.
- Using standard precautions whenever contact with blood, body fluids, secretions, excretions, mucous membranes, or nonintact skin is likely.

NURSING ASSISTANT ALERT

Action	Benefit
Provide emotional support by being calm, efficient, and a willing listener.	Builds patient confidence and helps reduce fears.
Carry out pre- and postoperative orders carefully.	Reduces the likelihood of postoperative complications.
Assemble necessary equipment and prepare the room for the patient's return from surgery.	Appropriate care can be immediately given as needed. Time is not wasted.
Observe the patient closely as postoperative exercise and ambulation are attempted. Be prepared to assist.	Avoids patient injury.
Report observations accurately and promptly.	Proper nursing interventions may be employed that promote recovery.

ACTIVITIES

Vocabulary Exercise

Complete the puzzle by filling in the missing letters of words found in this unit. Use the definitions to help you discover these words.

1. _ _ _ _ _ _ _ S _ _   1. Artificial body part

2.   _ _ _ U _ _ _ _ _ _   2. Walking

3.   _ _ R _ _ _ _   3. Dizziness

4.   _ _ _ G _ _ _ _ _   4. Hiccup

5.   _ _ _ _ _ I _ _   5. Sitting with feet over bed edge

6.   _ _ _ _ C _ _ _ _ _   6. Infection that develops in the hospital

7. _ _ _ _ _ _ _ A _ _ _   7. Collapse of lung tissue

8.   _ _ _ _ L _ _ _ _   8. Removes hair

Matching

Match each statement on the left with the correct word on the right.

1. _____ opening into the body
2. _____ the period following surgery
3. _____ drawing foreign material into the lungs
4. _____ lack of adequate oxygen supply
5. _____ loss of feeling or sensation
6. _____ inflammation of veins that can cause blood clots
7. _____ dizziness
8. _____ less than normal skin color
9. _____ difficulty breathing
10. _____ moving blood clot

a. embolus
b. dyspnea
c. pallor
d. singultus
e. orifice
f. vertigo
g. thrombophlebitis
h. postoperative
i. hypoxia
j. aspiration
k. anesthesia

Completion

Complete the following statements in the spaces provided.

1. The three phases of care required by the surgical patient are:

   a. _____

   b. _____

   c. _____

2. The purpose of anesthesia is _____.

3. Gaseous anesthetics are _____.

4. When patients have general anesthesia, they are apt to _____ postoperatively.

5. Gaseous anesthetics keep the patient _____ during surgery.

6. With a local anesthetic, the patient may remain _____ during surgery.

7. When a spinal anesthetic is given, all sensations _____ the level of the injection are _____.

8. Intravenous anesthetics make the patient fall asleep _____.

9. Seven duties the nursing assistant may be assigned in regard to the preoperative patient are:

   a. _____

   b. _____

   c. _____

   d. _____

   e. _____

   f. _____

   g. _____

10. Equipment left on the bedside table after the recovery bed is made includes:

    _____

11. When a patient vomits, his head should be _____ to prevent _____.

12. Spinal anesthesia is often given for abdominal surgery because it produces good

    _____

13. Patient questions should be referred to the _____.

14. The patient's position should be changed every _____ hours following surgery.

15. You should check the patient's _____ frequently as the patient dangles or ambulates for the first time.

16. Binders that are ordered postoperatively must be:

    a. _____

    b. _____

    c. _____

17. Elasticized stockings or Ace bandages are applied postoperatively to help support the _____ of the legs.

18. Postoperative leg exercises should be performed _____ times every _____ hours.

Complete the following statements regarding postoperative discomfort in the spaces provided.

19. The patient complains of thirst. You should give special _____ care and check for signs of _____.

20. The patient has singultus. You should support the _____ area.

21. The patient complains of pain. You should report the _____, _____, and _____ of pain.

22. The patient's abdomen is distended. You should encourage increased _____.

23. The patient has urinary retention. You should monitor _____ carefully.

24. The patient is hemorrhaging. You should keep the patient quiet and check _____

    _____

25. The patient may be going into shock. You suspect this because there is a fall in _____, the pulse is _____, the skin is _____, and the skin color is pale.

26. The patient is suffering from hypoxia. You should _____ to a sitting or _____ position and monitor oxygen if ordered.

27. The patient has suffered wound disruption. You should keep the patient _____ and _____ the incision area.

28. If a depilatory is used before surgery to remove hair, the nursing assistant should

    _____.

29. If the skin area to which a depilatory has been applied becomes reddened, the nursing assistant should

    _____.

30. If an electric clipper is used to prepare the operative area, the heads should be _____ or _____.

31. Identify each of the following items.

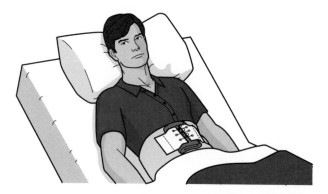

a. _____

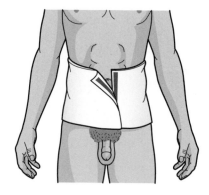

b. _____

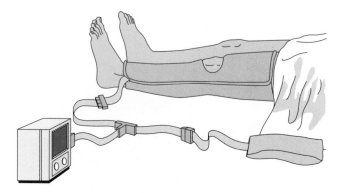

c. _____

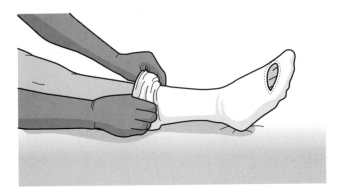

d. _____

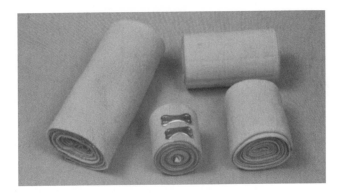

e. _____

32. State the name of each pulse.

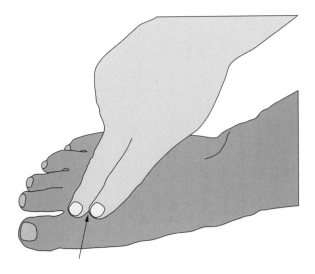

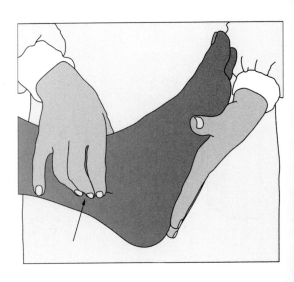

a. _____   b. _____

Short Answer

Answer the following questions.

1. What is needed for pain sensations to be realized?

   a. _____

   b. _____

   c. _____

2. What information is taught to the patient before surgery?

   a. _____

   b. _____

   c. _____

3. Why must nosocomial infections be prevented?

   a. _____

   b. _____

   c. _____

4. What actions should you take before the final preoperative medication is given?

   a. _____

   b. _____

   c. _____

   d. _____

   e. _____

   f. _____

   g. _____

5. What actions should you take after the medication is given?

   a. _____

   b. _____

   c. _____

   d. _____

   e. _____

6. What actions would you take while the patient is in the operating room?

   a. _____

   b. _____

   c. _____

7. What actions should be taken when the patient returns from surgery?

   a. _____

   b. _____

   c. _____

   d. _____

   e. _____

8. What special precautions should be taken when drainage tubes are in place?

   a. _____
   b. _____
   c. _____
   d. _____
   e. _____
   f. _____
   g. _____
   h. _____

9. Examine the following surgical checklist. List the items that are direct nursing assistant responsibilities.

   a. _____
   b. _____
   c. _____
   d. _____
   e. _____
   f. _____
   g. _____
   h. _____
   i. _____

> 1. Admission sheet
> 2. Surgical consent
> 3. Sterilization consent (if necessary)
> 4. Consultation sheet (if necessary)
> 5. History and physical
> 6. Lab reports (pregnancy tests also, if necessary)
> 7. Surgery prep done and charted, if required
> 8. Latest TPR and blood pressure charted
> 9. Preoperative medication given and charted (if required)
> 10. Wrist identification band on patient
> 11. Fingernail polish and makeup removed
> 12. Metallic objects removed (rings may be taped, if permitted)
> 13. Dentures removed
> 14. Other prostheses removed (such as artificial limb or eye)
> 15. Bath blanket and head cap in place
> 16. Bed in high position and side rails up after preop medication is given
> 17. Patient has voided

10. Define *perioperative hypothermia* and explain why it occurs. Describe what must happen before temperature stabilizes and approximately how long this takes. State the implications of this condition for nursing assistant care.

_____

_____

_____

_____

_____

11. Describe how to determine which size of anti-embolism hosiery should be used for the patient and explain why having the correct size is important.

_____

_____

_____

_____

True/False

Mark the following true or false by circling T or F.

1. T F Vital signs should be taken every 2 hours during the immediate postoperative period.
2. T F Many facilities view pain as the fifth vital sign.
3. T F Bandages are used to cover the wound.
4. T F Dressings are wrapped around bandages to hold them in place.
5. T F Montgomery straps are long adhesive strips with ties to hold dressings in place.
6. T F Sequential compression therapy is used to prevent blood clots.
7. T F Check the brachial and femoral pulses before applying pneumatic hosiery.
8. T F Pneumatic hosiery may be applied over anti-embolism hose.
9. T F Pneumatic hosiery should be removed every 6 hours for 30 minutes.
10. T F Deep vein thrombosis and pulmonary embolus (blood clot in the lungs) are serious postoperative complications.
11. T F Binders may be used to hold dressings in place.
12. T F Caring for wound drains involves the use of sterile technique.
13. T F The skin surrounding a drain is usually very red.
14. T F Empty chest drainage bottles once each shift.

Clinical Situations

Briefly describe how a nursing assistant should react to the following situations.

1. You are assigned to do a pubic prep and your patient's pubic hair is very long.

_____

_____

2. You are assisting a patient with initial ambulation, and the patient faints.

   _____

   _____

3. You find that the anti-embolism stockings your patient is wearing are wrinkled and have slipped down his leg.

   _____

   _____

4. Your postoperative patient's blood pressure has dropped and her pulse is rapid and weak. Her skin is cold and moist. _____

   _____

5. Your postoperative patient is anxious, has a feeling of heaviness in his chest, and is cyanotic.

   _____

   _____

RELATING TO THE NURSING PROCESS

Write the step of the nursing process that is related to the nursing assistant action.

Nursing Assistant Action   **Nursing Process Step**

1. The nursing assistant listens to and reports to the nurse the patient's concerns about scheduled surgery.   _____

2. The nursing assistant helps the patient bathe or shower with surgical soap.   _____

3. The nursing assistant checks with the nurse to determine the specific area to be shaved for surgery.   _____

4. Following shaving, the nursing assistant removes unattached hairs by gently pressing the sticky side of surgical tape against them.   _____

5. The nursing assistant makes sure there are no wrinkles in elasticized stockings once they are applied.   _____

6. The nursing assistant finds that the patient's pulse rate has increased more than 10 bpm after initial standing. The nursing assistant returns the patient to bed and reports to the nurse.   _____

DEVELOPING GREATER INSIGHT

1. Discuss ways you can assist a patient to support himself when he tries to cough and deep breathe following surgery.

2. Discuss ways you can contribute to the prevention of nosocomial infections.

3. With so many people having short-term surgery today, your contact with surgery patients may be limited. Think about ways you can make these contacts the most beneficial to the patient.

4. Optional: Your instructor will inform you if completing this figure is part of your assignment.

Surgical Prep Areas

Shade in the surgical prep areas that are to be shaved before surgery with colored pencil or crayon as indicated.

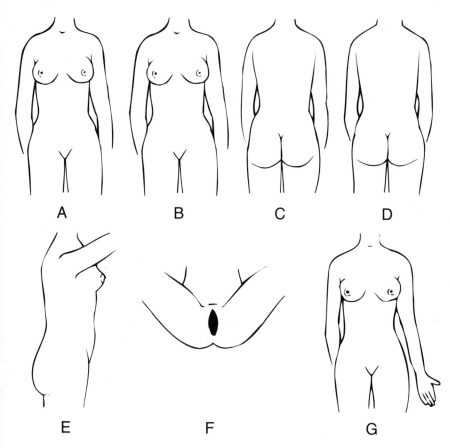

a. abdominal surgery

b. breast surgery—anterior

c. breast surgery—posterior

d. back surgery

e. kidney surgery

f. vaginal, rectal, and perineal surgery

Caring for the Emotionally Stressed Patient

After completing this unit, you will be able to:

- Spell and define terms.
- Define mental health and understand that it is a process of adaptations.
- Define affective disorders and describe bipolar affective disorder, schizoaffective disorder, seasonal affective disorder, borderline personality disorder, and depression.
- Give an overview of anorexia nervosa and bulimia nervosa.
- Explain how physical and mental health are related.
- Discuss substance abuse and describe the care of persons who are in withdrawal.
- Identify common defense mechanisms.
- Describe ways to help patients cope with stressful situations.
- Discuss mental illness and describe the care of persons with adaptive and maladaptive behavior.
- Describe methods of caring for the demanding patient.
- List at least 10 guidelines for dealing with a violent individual.
- Describe bullying behavior, identify triggers, and list steps to prevent being the target of a bully.

UNIT SUMMARY

Mental and physical health are interrelated. They influence the individual's ability to cope with life within the framework of society.

Mental health is maintained through the use of different coping mechanisms, such as:

- Repression
- Suppression
- Projection
- Denial

- Reaction formation
- Displacement
- Identification
- Compensation
- Conversion
- Undoing

Failure of coping mechanisms leads to maladaptive behaviors. These include:

- Excessive demands
- Alcoholism
- Depression
- Disorientation
- Agitation
- Anorexia nervosa, bulimia nervosa, and other eating disorders
- Anxiety and anxiety disorder
- Obsession

- Compulsions
- Panic disorder
- Phobia
- Posttraumatic stress disorder (PTSD)
- Paranoia
- Suicide attempts

The nursing assistant has specific responsibilities when caring for patients who exhibit maladaptive behaviors. These include:

- Observing and objectively reporting behaviors.
- Ensuring patient safety.
- Intervening in behaviors as directed by the care plan.
- Respecting professional boundaries with patients and families.
- Behaving in an ethical manner and avoiding personal relationships with patients and families.

NURSING ASSISTANT ALERT

Action	Benefit
Observe and objectively report patient behaviors.	Ensures correct evaluation.
Closely supervise patient activities.	Prevents patient injury.
Be consistent in your approach.	Helps patients reorient. Lessens the degree of confusion. Contributes to patient's sense of security.
Be vigilant in recognizing potentially unsafe situations.	Allows early interventions that reduce the likelihood of injury to patients or staff.

ACTIVITIES

Vocabulary Exercise

In the puzzle, find and circle each of the following words. In the space provided, define each word.

a	D	p	a	s	r	e	p	r	e	s	s	i	o	n	m	y	T	s	d
d	c	A	a	n	i	o	b	s	e	s	s	i	o	n	g	y	u	i	y
a	o	C	S	r	o	s	h	O	V	G	W	R	M	D	X	i	s	t	d
p	m	b	a	a	a	r	a	G	B	e	c	T	z	T	c	o	e	e	B
t	p	l	g	s	i	n	e	i	r	K	Y	W	u	i	r	i	n	z	d
a	u	V	i	t	G	b	o	x	r	n	e	Q	d	i	x	i	j	y	v
t	l	O	t	r	w	p	o	i	i	d	r	e	e	n	a	g	F	A	k
i	s	n	a	e	Y	c	U	h	a	a	n	n	a	l	I	W	y	R	s
o	i	o	t	s	r	e	W	u	p	R	t	O	e	H	R	A	G	I	n
n	o	i	i	s	Y	q	X	e	f	a	s	n	h	Z	E	C	s	F	o
W	n	t	o	o	O	l	e	O	t	u	a	V	a	c	W	I	t	z	i
G	k	c	n	r	z	a	w	i	p	b	y	T	C	i	o	X	u	M	s
j	o	e	c	s	z	G	o	p	I	U	x	S	a	g	m	p	p	I	u
H	x	j	y	G	Y	n	r	i	u	Y	O	S	D	p	n	i	y	i	l
s	o	o	o	s	p	e	n	s	k	h	C	w	p	F	I	i	l	h	e
o	Q	r	R	a	s	g	y	x	I	c	c	d	b	x	T	D	p	u	d
h	Y	p	n	s	Y	N	G	o	e	v	i	t	c	e	f	f	a	o	b
b	A	i	i	d	e	p	r	e	s	s	i	o	n	H	t	e	e	d	c
d	c	o	b	o	u	n	d	a	r	i	e	s	f	K	u	Y	J	a	Z
b	n	W	z	T	W	i	j	R	S	m	s	i	l	o	h	o	C	l	a

1. adaptation

   _____

2. affective

   _____

3. agitation

   _____

4. alcoholism

   _____

5. anorexia

   _____

6. anxiety

_____

7. bulimia

_____

8. compulsion

_____

9. coping

_____

10. delusions

_____

11. denial

_____

12. depression

_____

13. disorientation

_____

14. DT

_____

15. hypochondriasis

_____

16. obsession

_____

17. panic

_____

18. paranoia

_____

19. phobia

_____

20. projection

_____

21. repression

_____

22. SAD

_____

23. stressors

_____

24. suicide

_____

25. suppression

_____

Completion

Complete the following statements in the spaces provided.

1. Mental health means exhibiting behaviors that reflect a person's _____ to the multiple stresses of life.

2. A situation that makes a person anxious about his well-being is called a _____.

3. Poor mental health is demonstrated by _____.

4. Physical and mental health are _____.

5. A word used to mean handling stress is _____ with stress.

6. People use _____ mechanisms to protect their self-esteem.

7. Demanding patients are usually only expressing their own _____.

8. Some people turn to alcohol as a means of _____.

9. Alcohol _____ brain activity.

10. Alcohol is a drug that mixes _____ with other drugs.

11. Older alcoholics have a _____ chance of recovery.

12. The best approach to the disoriented patient is one that is _____ and _____.

13. Agitation is defined as inappropriate vocal or _____ activity due to causes other than confusion or need.

14. The patient who is disoriented may benefit from _____ orientation.

15. An extreme maladaptive response in which the person feels everyone is against him is called _____.

16. The nursing assistant must be sensitive to non _____ clues to the sources of a patient's stress.

17. It is important for the patient who is under stress to feel that the nursing assistant is _____ and will respect privacy and feelings.

18. Be supportive of the patient's own _____ to overcome the stress.

19. Patients often show their frustrations by being very _____.

20. A _____ is a purposeful, repetitive activity such as handwashing that is done many times each day and is beyond the person's control.

21. _____ is a condition in which the person has nightmares or flashbacks, and may have trouble with normal emotional responses. It is common in survivors of major trauma.

22. A _____ is an unfounded, recurring fear that causes the person to feel panic.

True/False

Mark the following true or false by circling T or F.

1. T F You can help patients cope with stress by being a good listener.

2. T F You should try to make patients see situations from your point of view.

3. T F It is all right to argue the point if you know the patient is wrong.

4. T F Panic attacks are mental illnesses involving anxiety reactions in response to stress.

5. T F Disorientation and depression may be associated with both physical and mental disorders.

6. T F The most common functional disorder in the geriatric age group is depression.

7. T F Some properly used drugs can cause a person to feel depressed.

8. T F A proper approach to the depressed patient is to let him know how sorry you feel for him.

9. T F The person who threatens suicide never attempts it.

10. T F An elderly person who has just lost a spouse is at risk for suicide.

11. T F The suicidal patient needs help in restoring her feelings of self-esteem.

12. T F Agitation is a significant problem for the elderly, their families, and the nursing staff.

13. T F The patient who is agitated has a prolonged attention span.

14. T F Constipation and dehydration can contribute to agitation.

15. T F One way to help the depressed patient is to reinforce his self-concept as a valued member of society.

16. T F The person who is depressed feels better if you express pity for her.

17. T F The disoriented person may show disorientation to time, person, or place.

18. T F Labeling a behavior implies passing judgment.

19. T F Speaking to others in the same way the supervisor speaks to you is a form of compensation.

20. T F OCD is one form of anxiety disorder.

21. T F PTSD most commonly occurs in children and young teens.

22. T F Panic attacks seldom recur.

23. T F A compulsion is a thought that makes no sense.

24. T F Phobias may cause a person to panic.

25. T F Snakes, spiders, and rats are common fears that may cause a person to feel panic.

26. T F Affective disorders are seldom characterized by a disturbance in mood.

27. T F Patients with bipolar disorder have mood swings ranging from elation to severe depression.

28. T F Patients with schizoaffective disorder may have delusions and hallucinations.

29. T F Patients with borderline personality disorder are often very manipulative.

30. T F People with BPD are often indecisive and prefer that others take charge.

31. T F One positive aspect of BPD is that persons with this condition usually maintain stable, long-term relationships.

32. T F Females with eating disorders may stop having menstrual periods.

33. T F Males do not develop eating disorders.

34. T F Males with some mental health conditions lose interest in sex.

35. T   F   Substance abuse may cause impaired judgment and maladaptive behavior.

36. T   F   Culture affects a person's feelings about mental illness.

37. T   F   The DTs usually occur when individuals withdraw from illegal drugs; they seldom occur as a result of use of substances such as alcohol, which can be legally purchased.

38. T   F   Suicide precautions are measures and practices a facility follows if a patient is at risk of harming himself or herself.

39. T   F   Suicide precautions are seldom necessary with persons who are mentally ill.

40. T   F   Signs and symptoms of delirium tremens include hallucinations and tremors.

41. T   F   Street names for methamphetamine include chocolate chip cookies, ice, and fizzies.

42. T   F   The effects of methadone are not always predictable.

Short Answer

Briefly answer the following questions.

1. List five common life stresses.

   a. _____

   b. _____

   c. _____

   d. _____

   e. _____

2. Explain each of the following defense mechanisms.

   a. projection _____

   _____

   b. denial _____

   _____

   c. identification _____

   _____

   d. fantasy _____

   _____

   e. compensation _____

   _____

3. List four ways to deal successfully with a demanding patient.

   a. _____

   b. _____

   c. _____

   d. _____

4. List five ways a nursing assistant can assist an alcoholic patient.

    a. _____

    b. _____

    c. _____

    d. _____

    e. _____

5. List five signs and symptoms indicating that a patient is depressed.

    a. _____

    b. _____

    c. _____

    d. _____

    e. _____

6. List eight signs and symptoms that indicate disorientation.

    a. _____

    b. _____

    c. _____

    d. _____

    e. _____

    f. _____

    g. _____

    h. _____

7. List six ways you can help a disoriented patient become better oriented to reality.

    a. _____

    b. _____

    c. _____

    d. _____

    e. _____

    f. _____

Clinical Situations

Briefly describe how a nursing assistant should react to the following situations.

1. Mrs. Sears has trouble sleeping, seems lethargic, and frequently dabs tears from her eyes.

    a. _____

    b. _____

    c. _____

2. Mr. Osborn is recovering from a head injury sustained in a fall downstairs. He insists that the patient in the next room is his daughter and tries to see her.

   a. _____

   b. _____

   c. _____

   d. _____

3. Mrs. Bell is pacing in the corridor. The nurse said in the report that she may be experiencing delirium. She repeatedly asks the same question to the staff. She sometimes bites and spits at others. Explain the factors that will contribute to her agitation.

   a. _____

   b. _____

   c. _____

   d. _____

   e. _____

   f. _____

   g. _____

   h. _____

RELATING TO THE NURSING PROCESS

Write the step of the nursing process that is related to the nursing assistant action.

Nursing Assistant Action   **Nursing Process Step**

1. The nursing assistant listens but does not argue even though the patient's belief is clearly wrong.   _____

2. The nursing assistant reports the patient's use of profanity without labeling his behavior.   _____

3. The nurse observes the way the patient says words and the body language she uses at the time.   _____

4. The nursing assistant reports to the nurse about ways he has found to help the patient deal with stress.   _____

5. The nursing assistant acts in a positive way when a patient is depressed.   _____

6. The nursing assistant reports that the patient is having crying spells.   _____

7. The nursing assistant gives instructions slowly and clearly, in simple words, to a disoriented person.   _____

DEVELOPING GREATER INSIGHT

1. Complete the chart to demonstrate your understanding of the concept of how people cope with stress. Discuss this with your classmates. Think carefully about your own coping mechanisms. Could you find more appropriate ways of dealing with stress?

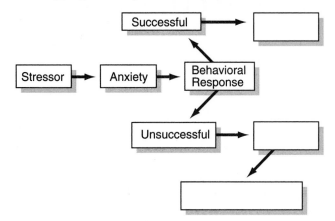

2. Look around your facility or clinical area. Try to identify anything that might be a safety hazard for a disoriented person.

3. Role-play with classmates the proper way to manage an agitated patient. Have one student act as the patient.

4. Think about your relationships with your teacher and classmates. Can you identify any situation in which you used one of the defense mechanisms described in this unit?

5. Discuss with the class ways you personally have found that help reduce stress.

Caring for the Bariatric Patient

OBJECTIVES

After completing this unit, you will be able to:

- Spell and define terms.
- Define overweight, obesity, and morbid obesity, and explain how these conditions differ from each other.
- Explain why weight affects lifespan (longevity) and health.
- Define comorbidities and explain how they affect a person's health.
- Briefly state how obesity affects the cardiovascular and respiratory systems.
- Explain how stereotyping and discrimination affect persons with obesity.
- List some team members and their responsibilities in the care of the bariatric patient.
- Explain why environmental modifications are needed for bariatric patient care.
- Describe observations to make and methods of meeting bariatric patients' ADL needs.
- List precautions to take when moving and positioning bariatric patients.
- List at least five complications of immobility in bariatric patients.
- Describe nursing assistant responsibilities in the postoperative care of patients who have had bariatric surgery.

UNIT SUMMARY

The incidence of overweight and obesity is increasing in the United States, affecting about one in three adults. The rise in obesity has been rapid in children. As a result, more patients with these conditions are being admitted to the hospital, and staff must know how to safely care for them and meet their unique needs.

Some patients will be admitted for medical problems; others are admitted for bariatric surgery. Comorbidities must be treated and stabilized before surgery can be done. A team effort is essential to good patient care.

- Obesity has many causes, including heredity.

212

- Body mass index (BMI) is a mathematical calculation used to determine whether a person is at a healthy, normal weight; is overweight; or is obese.

- Obesity is usually defined as being overweight by 20 to 30 percent of the ideal body weight.

- Obesity negatively affects every body system, increases the risk for other serious medical problems, and results in a shorter lifespan if untreated.

- Persons with obesity experience discrimination and prejudice, difficulty in ADLs, and limited access to public facilities. They may also have relationship difficulties or be victims of physical and psychological abuse. When they are hospitalized, they know that their size makes it hard for staff to care for them, and they may be admitted to your unit with feelings of shame, embarrassment, and fear.

- Supporting patients' dignity and self-esteem is of critical importance.

- Bariatrics is a relatively new field of medicine that focuses on the treatment and control of obesity and medical conditions and diseases associated with obesity.

- Environmental modifications and special equipment and supplies are needed in the care of bariatric patients. Essential equipment and supply items are bariatric:

  ○ Hospital gowns

  ○ Blood pressure cuffs or other devices for measuring blood pressure

  ○ Beds

  ○ Scales

  ○ Toilets or commodes

  ○ Electrical or mechanical lifts and equipment to facilitate transfers

  ○ Room furnishings

- Nursing assistants must keep patient and personal safety in mind when caring for bariatric patients. Situations for which the assistant may need special equipment and/or additional help are:

  ○ Moving and positioning the patient.

  ○ Assisting with ADLs and toileting.

  ○ Mobility and ambulation.

- The skin is the largest organ of the body; the skin of the bariatric patient usually has been stretched and is easily injured. Provide care to prevent injury from moisture, pressure, friction, and shear force.

- Bariatric patients are at very high risk of complications when they are immobile. Those who are unconscious or bedfast are at high risk of developing:

  ○ Pneumonia

  ○ Atelectasis

  ○ Deep vein thrombosis (blood clots in the legs)

  ○ Pulmonary embolism (blood clot in the lungs)

  ○ Pressure ulcers

  ○ Yeast infections in the skin folds

NURSING ASSISTANT ALERT

Action	Benefit
Attend continuing education classes to learn how to meet the physical and emotional care needs of the bariatric patient.	Expand your nursing assistant knowledge for personal benefit and to meet the needs of a new patient population.
Become familiar with bariatric equipment and how to use it.	Ensures nursing assistant and patient safety.
Monitor for and report potential risk factors, complications, and unsafe situations.	Ensures timely assessment and intervention to improve patient outcomes.
Meet patients' emotional and psychosocial needs through empathy, sensitivity, and compassionate caring.	Promotes patient satisfaction with care and enhances self-esteem.

Provide pre- and postoperative care to the patient undergoing bariatric surgery; be familiar with, monitor for, and report complications.

Monitor for and actively provide nursing care to reduce risk factors and prevent complications of immobility.

Decreases preoperative anxiety.
Reduces strain on staples postoperatively.
Helps ensure that potential complications are promptly assessed and treated.

Enhances patient confidence and comfort.
Helps eliminate complications and comorbidities.

Vocabulary Exercise

1. Find the following words in the puzzle. *Words in parentheses are not in the puzzle.* In the space provided, write a definition of each word.

q	f	t	h	t	r	a	p	e	z	e	o	x	w	O	p	h	n	a	i
p	u	e	h	y	T	d	A	d	X	y	G	H	I	c	I	M	B	n	e
p	O	o	r	g	p	M	H	Y	U	z	o	p	H	k	t	z	v	t	I
f	J	b	m	u	i	e	U	m	Y	t	V	V	H	R	c	a	a	S	s
X	m	e	o	t	t	e	r	f	J	t	O	X	A	x	s	c	M	e	n
m	r	s	r	R	H	c	w	v	x	z	U	N	S	i	o	h	i	e	f
i	T	i	b	H	F	e	i	r	e	y	e	Q	v	v	o	t	M	g	K
k	c	t	i	x	a	r	F	r	e	n	z	e	d	w	i	M	i	t	C
n	i	y	d	I	P	q	R	r	t	v	t	a	U	d	x	e	R	X	b
o	p	c	Z	A	A	Y	w	u	V	s	o	i	i	T	S	A	q	p	V
i	o	x	B	N	D	a	J	d	V	p	s	b	I	g	k	L	C	a	t
s	c	d	p	Q	w	q	d	J	a	c	r	s	a	a	d	C	f	i	d
n	s	D	b	p	F	j	y	n	i	o	p	n	e	d	t	x	y	d	x
e	o	F	u	X	f	k	n	r	m	l	i	O	k	t	D	i	a	D	u
t	r	o	L	O	k	i	t	o	C	U	d	O	W	X	e	w	o	U	I
r	a	Z	b	S	c	a	c	s	f	E	p	E	Z	d	o	b	w	n	f
e	p	B	p	u	i	j	g	E	G	T	I	M	C	I	V	o	a	F	e
p	a	h	I	r	I	B	W	M	C	o	j	P	V	j	N	y	f	i	r
y	I	u	a	b	y	p	a	s	s	E	F	e	w	k	o	n	k	z	d
h	s	b	v	g	T	b	I	y	O	P	Y	s	i	s	o	n	e	t	s

a. advocate

_____

b. bariatrics

_____

c. BMI

_____

d. comorbidities

_____

e. diabetes

_____

f. (gastric) bypass

_____

g. hypertension

_____

h. hyperventilation

_____

i. IBW

_____

j. (minimally) invasive (surgery)

_____

k. laparoscopic

_____

l. morbid (obesity)

_____

m. obesity

_____

n. overweight

_____

o. panniculus

_____

p. reflux

_____

q. stenosis

_____

r. stricture

_____

s. trapeze

_____

True/False

Mark the following true or false by circling T or F.

1. T   F   A person who is overweight has a BMI over 50.
2. T   F   Most obese people eat an enormous amount of food and lack willpower.
3. T   F   Obesity negatively affects every system of the body.
4. T   F   Obesity is commonly hereditary; environmental factors have no effect on weight.
5. T   F   Obesity is considered a chronic condition.
6. T   F   A fat baby is a healthy baby.

7.   T   F   The BMI is diagnostic of an individual's health status.

8.   T   F   Comorbidities are diseases and medical conditions that are either caused by or contributed by morbid obesity.

9.   T   F   Persons with obesity are at increased risk for cancer.

10.   T   F   Adipose tissue is poorly nourished and less resistant to injury than the tissues of a smaller person.

11.   T   F   The weight of an obese person's chest makes breathing more difficult.

12.   T   F   The bariatric nurse specialist writes the dietary plan of care and supervises the menu.

13.   T   F   The bariatric patient cannot develop malnutrition or dehydration because of the nutrient stores in the adipose tissue.

14.   T   F   Bariatric patients often sweat profusely.

15.   T   F   Gore-Tex and nylon sheets have a slippery surface that reduces friction and shear and makes it easier to move the patient.

16.   T   F   If the patient is too large for the regular scale, obtain the freight scale or laundry scale from the maintenance department.

17.   T   F   The patient advocate's main responsibility is protecting the bariatric patient's dignity.

18.   T   F   Do not ask the patient what works for his or her care, because it will appear that you do not know what you are doing.

19.   T   F   A regular washcloth and towel may be very irritating to the skin of some bariatric patients.

20.   T   F   Bariatric patients may need extra fluids to support their body needs.

21.   T   F   A condom catheter is commonly used for male bariatric patients because it is easier than inserting a regular catheter, stays in place well, and requires less frequent peri care.

22.   T   F   Bariatric patients seldom develop pressure ulcers because of the extra padding over bony prominences.

23.   T   F   One staff person should never lift or move more than 55 pounds of body weight without extra help or a mechanical device.

24.   T   F   Two or more nursing assistants are often needed to assist the bariatric patient with personal hygiene procedures.

25.   T   F   Using the Trendelenburg position when moving the bariatric patient up in bed makes the job easier and reduces the risk of injury.

Short Answer

Briefly answer the following questions.

1. When the patient is positioned on his or her side, you should _____

_____

2. Why does the obese patient walk with a wide-based gait? _____

_____

3. The nurse may instruct you to apply an abdominal binder before moving the bariatric patient. Why is this done?

_____

_____

4. If a standing bariatric patient begins to fall to the floor, what is the most important action to take?

_____

_____

_____

5. Identify the three most common complications of bariatric surgery.

   a. _____

   b. _____

   c. _____

6. What is the primary goal of the postoperative care given to a person who has had bariatric surgery?

_____

_____

_____

7. Explain why the patient is permitted to have only very small amounts of food or fluid after bariatric surgery.

_____

_____

_____

8. List at least five potentially serious signs and symptoms of postoperative complications that should be reported to the nurse promptly.

_____

_____

_____

_____

_____

9. Identify this item and describe why it is used.

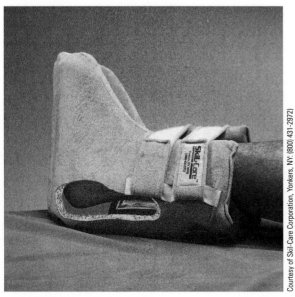

Courtesy of Skil-Care Corporation, Yonkers, NY. (800) 431-2972)

10. Identify this item and describe when it should be used.

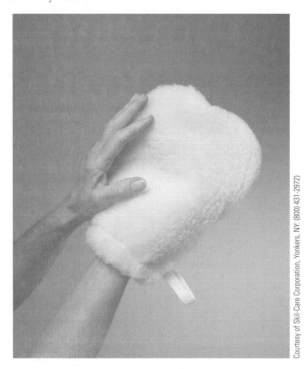

Courtesy of Skil-Care Corporation, Yonkers, NY: (800) 431-2972)

_____

RELATING TO THE NURSING PROCESS

Write the step of the nursing process that is related to the nursing assistant action.

Nursing Assistant Action   **Nursing Process Step**

1. The nursing assistant finds that the patient's blood pressure
   is 180/106, so she rechecks it. Finding the value the same,
   she seeks out the nurse to report her findings.   _____

2. The nurse has given Mr. Mulvaney an insulin injection.
   He instructs the nursing assistant to monitor for signs
   of hypoglycemia, to recheck the blood sugar in
   2 hours, and to report the value.   _____

3. Mr. Romcevich's plan of care is not working and the
   patient is dissatisfied. The nurse asks the nursing
   assistant about care plan approaches that have been
   effective, and which approaches have not worked.   _____

4. The nursing assistant notifies the nurse that Mr. Turpel,
   a recent bariatric surgery patient, is vomiting.   _____

5. The nursing assistant gets another assistant to help her
   perform peri care on Mrs. Evert.   _____

DEVELOPING GREATER INSIGHT

1. Think carefully about obese people you have known or seen in public. Identify problems and needs that normal-sized individuals do not experience. List as many as you can and report them to the class.

2. Patients often view the day of their bariatric surgery as the first day of the rest of their lives. Why do you think this is?

3. Why should you avoid making unsolicited comments, such as "you don't look like you need this (weight loss) surgery" or "but you really do carry your weight well"? Think carefully about your answer and report your findings to the class. What can we learn from this?

Death and Dying

OBJECTIVES

After completing this unit, you will be able to:

- Spell and define terms.
- Discuss the five stages of grief.
- Describe differences in how people handle the process of death and dying.
- Describe the spiritual preparations for death practiced by various religions.
- State the purpose of the Patient Self-Determination Act.
- Discuss Physician Orders for Life-Sustaining Treatment (POLST).
- Describe the nursing assistant's responsibilities for providing supportive care.
- Describe the hospice philosophy and method of care.
- List the signs of approaching death.
- Demonstrate the following procedure:

  Procedure 87   Giving Postmortem Care

UNIT SUMMARY

- Assisting with terminal and postmortem care is a difficult but essential part of nursing assistant duties. It requires a high degree of sensitivity, understanding, and tact.

- Both the patient and the family require support during this trying period.

- Care must be taken to provide for the religious preferences and cultural practices of the patient and the family.

- The procedure for postmortem care must be carried out with efficiency and respect.

NURSING ASSISTANT ALERT

Action	Benefit
Recognize that the stages of grief are experienced by both patient and family.	Allows staff to provide essential emotional support.
Remember that people react to a terminal diagnosis in a variety of ways.	Permits nursing care to be individualized.
Identify the signs of impending death.	Allows proper nursing care interventions to be carried out.
Treat the body with the same respect as the living patient.	Maintains dignity and respect.

ACTIVITIES

Vocabulary Exercise

Each line has four different spellings of a word. Circle the correctly spelled word.

1. critical	cretical	critecal	creticale
2. posmortum	postmartem	postmortem	postmortom
3. hopice	hopise	hospise	hospice
4. terminale	terminal	termanel	termanal
5. danial	deniel	denial	deniale
6. morabund	moribund	moreband	moribond
7. annointing	anointing	annointen	anontin
8. awtopsie	awtopsy	autopse	autopsy
9. bargaining	bargenan	bargainin	bergaining
10. rigor mortis	rigor mortus	rigger mortis	regor mortos

Completion

Complete the statements in the spaces provided.

1. When the patient's condition is critical, the _____ places the patient's name on the critical list.

2. Sacrament of the Sick is requested for the patient of the _____ faith.

3. Hospice care is based on the philosophy that death is a _____ process.

4. Hospice care is provided for people with a life expectancy of _____.

5. Hospice care is provided by _____ who work with the patient and the family.

6. As death approaches, body functions _____.

7. The last sense lost is the sense of _____.

8. As death approaches, the pulse becomes _____ and progressively _____.

9. The time of death is determined by the _____.

10. Under no circumstances should the _____ inform the family of the patient's death.

11. As a nursing assistant, you have a unique opportunity to be a source of _____ and _____ to the dying patient and the family.

12. During the dying period, you must provide the family and patient with _____.

13. The nursing assistant must realize that dying is a _____ each person must make _____.

True/False

Mark the following true or false by circling T or F.

1. T F A patient goes through each stage of grieving in a sequential order.

2. T F Once he or she has moved on to another stage of the grieving process, the patient never returns to a former stage.

3. T F All patients go through each stage of grieving at the same rate.

4. T F The nursing assistant must have an understanding attitude during each stage of the grieving process.

5. T F The family members may go through the same five stages of the grieving process.

6. T F The nursing assistant should reflect the patient's statements during the stage of denial.

7. T F If the patient seems depressed, it is best to leave him alone to work it out himself.

8. T F The patient in the stage of acceptance has no fear.

9. T F The stage of depression is often filled with expression of regrets.

10. T F The patient who has reached the stage of acceptance may try to assist those around her to deal with her death.

11. T F The Patient Self-Determination Act goes into effect as soon as a patient is admitted to a health care facility.

12. T F Supportive care for terminally ill patients does not include life-sustaining treatments.

13. T F The POLST document must be revised each time the patient's location changes.

14. T F The POLST document does not affect the advance directive.

Short Answer

Briefly answer the following questions in the spaces provided.

1. List the five stages of grief as outlined by E. Kübler-Ross.

   a. _____

   b. _____

   c. _____

   d. _____

   e. _____

2. What are the goals of hospice programs?

   a. _____

   b. _____

   c. _____

3. As a member of the hospice team, how can you promote the hospice philosophy?

   a. _____

   b. _____

   c. _____

   d. _____

4. What are five moribund changes?

   a. _____

   b. _____

   c. _____

   d. _____

   e. _____

5. What items would you expect to find in a morgue kit?

   a. _____

   b. _____

   c. _____

   d. _____

   e. _____

6. What should you do before moving the body to the morgue, to prevent upsetting other patients?

   _____

   _____

7. Why is the use of standard precautions necessary when performing postmortem care?

   _____

   _____

Clinical Situations

Briefly describe how a nursing assistant should react to the following situations.

1. Your terminal patient, who had been crying earlier, suddenly appears cheerful and talks about a trip he is planning for next year.

   _____

   _____

2. The patient expresses a desire to see her clergyperson.

   _____

3. The physician has pronounced the patient deceased and you are to prepare the patient for the return of the family.

   a. _____

   b. _____

   c. _____

   d. _____

   e. _____

4. The patient has an order for supportive care only. What care does this include?

   a. _____

   b. _____

   c. _____

   d. _____

5. The patient has both a living will and a durable power of attorney. Write the name of the document that assigns responsibility for handling the patient's personal affairs and making health care decisions for the patient.

   _____

6. A patient has a no-code order. State how this order influences care if the patient experiences respiratory and cardiac arrest.

   _____

RELATING TO THE NURSING PROCESS

Write the step of the nursing process that is related to the nursing assistant action.

Nursing Assistant Action	Nursing Process Step
1. The nursing assistant promptly reports complaints of pain by the terminally ill patient to the nurse.	_____
2. During the postmortem period, the nursing assistant cares for the body with dignity.	_____
3. The nursing assistant checks the dying patient frequently.	_____
4. The nursing assistant offers quiet support to the family of the dying patient by listening.	_____

DEVELOPING GREATER INSIGHT

1. Share with classmates any special traditions or practices that your family carries out when someone dies.

2. Invite members of different faiths to share some of their experiences with dying people.

3. Invite a nursing assistant or nurse who works in a hospice to come and share some of his or her experiences with the class.

4. Think how you might feel if you were giving care to a patient who is terminally ill and has an order for supportive care only.

Other Health Care Settings

Providing Care for Special Populations: Elderly, Chronically Ill, Alzheimer's Disease, Intellectual Disabilities, and Developmental Disabilities

OBJECTIVES

After completing this unit, you will be able to:

- Spell and define terms.
- Describe the services provided by the various types of long-term care facilities, and discuss how culture change is transforming long-term care services.
- Identify the expected changes of aging.
- Identify residents who are at risk for malnutrition and dehydration and list measures to promote sufficient intake.

- Discuss how to meet the hygiene and grooming needs of long-term care residents.

- Give an overview of at least eight diseases that cause dementia.

- Identify the three main stages of Alzheimer's disease and briefly describe each stage.

- Define delirium, explain how it differs from dementia, and list potential signs and symptoms to report.

- Describe the nursing assistant care for persons with cognitive impairment, disorientation, dementia, and wandering.

- State the purpose of animal-assisted therapy, music therapy, reality orientation, reminiscing, and validation therapy.

- List three criteria that must be present for a developmental disability diagnosis.

- Define intellectual disability and discuss the care of persons with this disorder and other common developmental disabilities.

- State the difference between a congenital developmental disability and an acquired developmental disability and give examples of each.

- Describe nursing assistant care and communication guidelines for persons with developmental disabilities.

UNIT SUMMARY

The person being cared for in the long-term health care facility:

- Is usually a mature adult.

- Often is elderly.

- Frequently has chronic and/or debilitating conditions.

Adult life spans a period of 50 years or more.

Basic care will be provided using the same techniques employed in the acute setting. Adaptations must be made because of the greater dependency of this group of residents. Physical changes occur in each body system as aging progresses.

It is important for the nursing assistant to remember that each person is a unique individual and must be treated with respect and dignity.

Adjustments to the aging process must be made on both physical and emotional levels. The nursing assistant can be a valuable source of caring and support. Special care needs have to be met in the following areas:

- Promoting patients' and residents' rights.

- Respecting spiritual needs.

- Maintaining personal hygiene.

- Assisting patients and residents with food and fluid intake and meeting dietary requirements.

- Ensuring adequate exercise.
- Caring for elimination.
- Meeting recreational needs.
- Supporting emotional adjustments.
- Orienting to reality.
- Providing a safe environment.
- Providing opportunities for social interactions.
- Preventing infections.

Culture-change facilities practice person-directed care. The facility is changed from a clinical environment into a comfortable, restraint-free, home-like community, in which residents are treated with respect.

Dementia is a disease of the brain cells and is not normal aging. It cannot be cured. Alzheimer's disease is the most common type of dementia. Despite having a healthy appearance, persons with dementia have changes in the structure and function of the brain. Nursing assistants are responsible for keeping all residents, including those with dementia, safe and assisting them to maintain their highest level of function for as long as possible.

Persons with intellectual disability (mental retardation) have lower-than-average intelligence, limited ability to learn, social immaturity, and a reduced ability to adapt to their environment. Persons who have a developmental disability developed the condition before the age of 22. Some have below-average intelligence, but many are of normal intelligence or above. The goal of care is to help these residents function at their maximum potential.

The nursing assistant works closely with facility patients or residents and is in a position to make observations regarding changes in their usual condition. Observation and reporting of changes in condition, which are frequently subtle, is a major responsibility.

Basic care and observations must be documented each day.

NURSING ASSISTANT ALERT

Action	Benefit
Familiarize yourself with the usual signs of aging.	Forms a baseline of comparison for abnormal findings.
Avoid stereotypes.	Encourages people to be seen as individuals.
Expect major adjustments when people are admitted to long-term care.	Interventions can be planned to reduce resident stress and anxiety.
Address each basic human need.	All aspects of the resident's human needs will be recognized and met through appropriate planning of nursing care.
Identify communication limitations and report them.	Interventions can be developed to improve the free flow of interactions.

ACTIVITIES

Vocabulary Exercise

Complete the crossword puzzle by using the definitions presented.

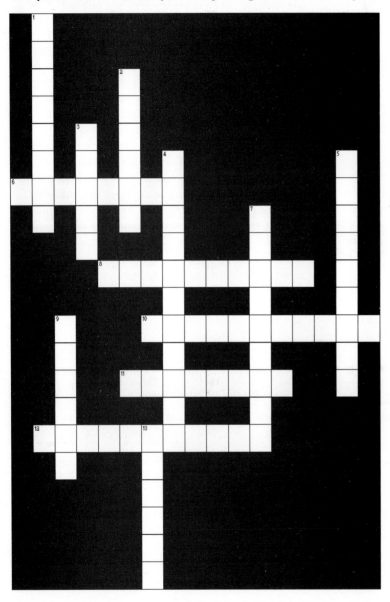

Across

6 Living actively, having adequate energy

8 Passing gas

10 Recalling past events

11 Disorder of the brain involving thinking, memory, and judgment

12 Encourage and provide sufficient fluids to prevent _____

Down

1 Excessive urination at night

2 Having an abnormally low body temperature is a common sign of a serious infection, called
   _____

3 Outcomes

4 Temperature below 95°F or cold relative to the resident's baseline temperature

5 Name given to people living in long-term care facilities

7 Relating to the teeth

9 Long-term care residents must cope with many _____

13 The regurgitation of stomach contents back into the esophagus

Definitions

Define the following words.

1. Medicaid _____

2. Pigmentation _____

3. Debilitating _____

4. Assisted living _____

5. Sundowning _____

6. Reminiscing _____

7. Diverticulitis _____

8. Chronological _____

9. Dementia _____

10. Long-term care _____

Matching

Match the words on the right with the statements on the left.

1. _____ capacity for endurance, having energy, living actively

2. _____ excessive gas in stomach or intestines

3. _____ condition in which a person has 47 chromosomes

4. _____ weakening

5. _____ craving to eat nonfood items

6. _____ genetic disorder caused by mutation in the RNA

7. _____ results from lack of oxygen during labor and delivery

8. _____ condition in which fluid applies pressure to the brain

9. _____ involuntary urination or defecation

10. _____ rate at which an illness occurs in a given population

11. _____ weakened places in intestinal wall

a. pica

b. cerebral palsy

c. hydrocephalus

d. vitality

e. morbidity

f. diverticula

g. debilitating

h. Fragile X

i. Down syndrome

j. flatulence

k. incontinence

Match the problem with the system affected.

1. _____ blood vessels less elastic

2. _____ constipation

3. _____ incontinence

4. _____ less flexibility

5. _____ diminished hearing

6. _____ decreased primary taste sensation

7. _____ flatulence

8. _____ slower movements

9. _____ diminished depth perception

10. _____ loss of hair color

a. integumentary

b. nervous

c. musculoskeletal

d. urinary

e. digestive

f. cardiovascular

True/False

Determine which of the following are true statements about all elderly people.

1. T   F   They no longer contribute to society.

2. T   F   They have no interest in sex.

3. T   F   They are living in poverty.

4. T   F   They have sensory losses.

5. T   F   They are incompetent to make decisions.

6. T   F   They have short-term memory loss.

7. T   F   They undergo postural changes.

8. T   F   They are more prone to certain chronic conditions.

9. T   F   They have changed sleep patterns.

10. T   F   They are unable to learn.

11. T   F   They have the same rights as any citizen of the United States.

Completion

Complete the following statements in the spaces provided.

1. To be successful as a long-term care nursing assistant, you must have a sense of _____ and be able to _____ effectively.

2. Every resident must be treated with _____.

3. Most of the residents in long-term care are _____ and have _____ health problems.

4. The long-term care nursing assistant must be satisfied with _____ progress and _____ gains.

5. Each person moves from infancy to old age at an _____ rate.

6. Some researchers believe that each person has an inborn biological _____.

7. Smell receptors and taste buds _____ with age.

8. Elderly people may not be _____ of their need for fluid.

9. Poor dental care and oral hygiene can result in loss of appetite and _____.

10. _____ maintains dignity by acknowledging memories and feelings.

11. Residents can and do develop _____, despite being served a balanced diet and having nutritional supplements available.

12. _____ is the most common type of dementia.

13. _____ is an acute confusional state caused by reversible medical problems.

14. Prion diseases are rapidly _____ and _____.

15. Another term for wandering away from the facility is _____.

16. Confused residents are very sensitive to the moods and _____ of staff members.

17. Seeing items associated with going outdoors may _____ wandering.

18. OBRA requires all nursing assistants working in long-term care to complete a course of at least _____ clock hours.

19. Competency tests may be taken _____ times.

20. Nursing assistants must take part in ongoing _____ education.

21. State certification lapses if the nursing assistant does not work for pay during any given _____ period of time.

22. Persons with _____ repeat their actions or words.

23. Frustrations at physical _____ and loss of _____ control are common among the elderly.

24. Elderly people may develop an apathy about food that results in _____.

25. Lotions should be applied to _____ dry skin.

26. A _____ is the response of a person with dementia to overwhelming stimuli.

Short Answer

Briefly answer the following questions in the space provided.

1. What are five changes frequently seen in the integumentary system of the elderly?

   a. _____
   b. _____
   c. _____
   d. _____
   e. _____

2. What are the four basic emotional needs of the elderly?

   a. _____
   b. _____
   c. _____
   d. _____

3. List the "fatal four" risks that are more common in people with developmental disabilities than in the general population.

    a. _____

    b. _____

    c. _____

    d. _____

4. Residents who are at greatest risk of malnutrition and unintentional weight loss are those who:

    a. _____

    b. _____

    c. _____

    d. _____

    e. _____

5. List five risks associated with pica.

    a. _____

    b. _____

    c. _____

    d. _____

    e. _____

6. What is meant by a "catastrophic reaction" relating to a person with dementia?

    _____

    _____

7. List five observations to make and report related to behavioral problems.

    a. _____

    b. _____

    c. _____

    d. _____

    e. _____

8. List five triggers of wandering.

    a. _____

    b. _____

    c. _____

    d. _____

    e. _____

True/False

Mark the following true or false by circling T or F.

1. T   F   Reminiscing is an inappropriate activity for elderly people.

2. T   F   Reminiscing helps people adapt to old age by allowing them to work through personal losses.

3. T   F   Reminiscing is a natural activity for people of all ages.

4. T   F   Reminiscing should be ignored because such remembrances have little relationship to today.

5. T   F   Clocks with large numbers should be placed around the facility.

6. T   F   Care for disoriented residents includes frequently asking residents to identify the date or the caregiver.

7. T   F   Treat adult residents as children when they act confused.

8. T   F   Call residents by cute or pet names so they will feel comfortable and at home.

9. T   F   Try to reason with the resident who is having a catastrophic reaction.

Multiple Choice

Select the one best answer for each of the following.

1. Skilled nursing care facilities:

    a. provide only assistance with activities of daily living.

    b. care only for acutely ill residents.

    c. provide care to residents with chronic conditions.

    d. employ only registered nurses.

2. Most residents in long-term care facilities:

    a. experience sundowning in the afternoon.

    b. have temporary acute conditions.

    c. require very little health care and supervision.

    d. have chronic, progressive conditions.

3. Which of the following applies to bathing the elderly?

    a. Full daily baths are essential.

    b. Bathing two to three times a week is fine.

    c. Frequent bathing is important.

    d. Use deodorants liberally.

4. Which of the following is true of nail care?

    a. Residents should never have dirty nails.

    b. Use a very stiff brush to clean nails.

    c. Clip fingernails at least once a week.

    d. Clean nails with a metal file.

5. A congenital condition:

   a. is acquired as a result of an accident.

   b. is present at the time of birth.

   c. develops between the ages of 8 and 22.

   d. results from lack of oxygen at birth.

6. Animal-assisted therapy has been shown to:

   a. relieve headache.

   b. cause agitation.

   c. reduce the incidence of allergies.

   d. lower blood pressure.

Clinical Situations

Briefly describe how a nursing assistant should react to the following situations.

1. Mrs. Li, age 92, is withdrawn much of the time but occasionally is complaining, hostile, and demanding. Her family seldom visits, and her behavior is the same toward them.

   _____

   _____

   _____

   _____

2. Mrs. Preston reported drinking a lot of water, but the water carafe was still almost full.

   _____

   _____

   _____

   _____

3. Mrs. Gutierrez keeps trying to leave the facility and insists that she must hurry home to cook dinner for the children.

   _____

   _____

   _____

   _____

Hidden Picture

Identify the problems that require attention in the picture.

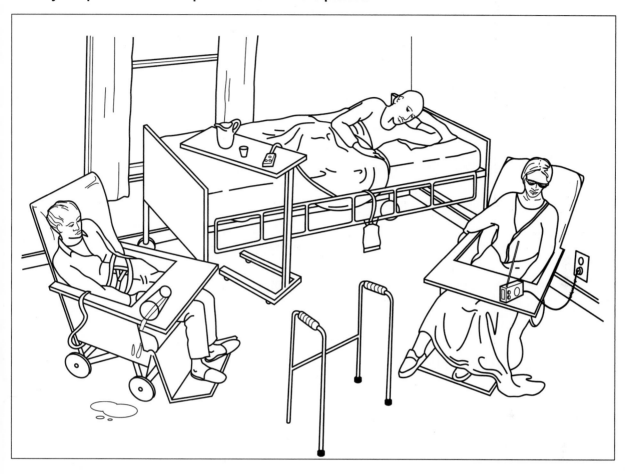

1. _____
2. _____
3. _____
4. _____
5. _____
6. _____
7. _____
8. _____

RELATING TO THE NURSING PROCESS

Write the step of the nursing process that is related to the nursing assistant action.

Nursing Assistant Action	Nursing Process Step
1. The nursing assistant reassures the people in his care that they will not be abandoned.	_____
2. The nursing assistant treats each resident with respect.	_____
3. The nursing assistant reports that the resident has complained of feeling constipated.	_____
4. The nursing assistant encourages the resident to feed himself but is ready to assist if needed.	_____
5. The nursing assistant encourages the resident to drink fluids frequently.	_____
6. The nursing assistant patiently works with the intellectually disabled resident to meet her care plan goal.	_____
7. The nursing assistant uses gestures to help communicate meaning when the resident has a hearing impairment.	_____

DEVELOPING GREATER INSIGHT

1. Discuss with classmates the differences between reality orientation and validation therapy, including how each is appropriately used and the possible benefits to residents.

2. Explain ways to protect the resident who wanders.

The Organization of Home Care: Trends in Health Care

OBJECTIVES

After completing this unit, you will be able to:

- Spell and define terms.
- Briefly outline the history of home care.
- Describe the types of nursing services that are provided in the home.
- Describe the benefits of working in home care.
- List the qualifications for working as a nursing assistant in home care.
- Identify members of the home health team.
- State the purpose of the case manager.
- State the purpose of the Outcome and Assessment Information Set (OASIS).
- List guidelines for avoiding liability while working as a home health assistant.
- Describe the types of information a home health assistant must be able to document.
- Identify several time management techniques.
- List ways in which the home health assistant can work successfully with client's families.

UNIT SUMMARY

There is an increasing trend to provide home health care to housebound, recuperating, and chronically ill patients, who are called *clients*. Home health care consists of:

- Maintaining a safe, comfortable environment for the client.
- Managing infection control.

- Carrying out proper nursing techniques under the supervision of the nurse case manager.

The home health assistant occupies the positions of:

- Member of the home health care team.
- Guest in the client's home.
- Provider of direct health care and household assistance.

237

NURSING ASSISTANT ALERT

Action	Benefit
Document according to agency policy.	Provides accurate information regarding caregiver, client progress, and financial costs.
Know the agency's nursing assistant job description and carry out those responsibilities only.	Avoids liability and assures cost reimbursement.
Know and support client's rights.	Assures that the client will be treated with respect and dignity.

ACTIVITIES

Vocabulary Exercise

Write the definition for each of the following.

1. Client care records _____

2. Intermittent care _____

3. Time/travel records _____

Completion

Complete the following statements in the spaces provided. Select the correct term from the list provided.

accuracy	assistance	calculations	complete
developed	home health care team	hospital	independence
insurance group	number	nurse	one
part-time	records	skilled nursing facility	taught

1. An advantage to working as a nursing assistant in the home is that there are opportunities for _____ employment.

2. In home care, there is the opportunity to give _____ care to _____ client at a time.

3. The home health care assistant has an opportunity to work with greater _____.

4. The care of the client is planned by the _____.

5. The services of the home nursing assistant may be implemented after a referral from a/an _____

6. It is important to keep accurate time and cost _____ of the care you give.

7. Most persons using home care have been discharged from a/an _____ or _____

8. Clients may be in need of _____ with activities of daily living.

9. A nursing assistant may be assigned to care for a client for a _____ of hours daily.

10. The care plan is _____ with the client by the _____.

11. Liability can be avoided if the nursing assistant carries out actions as he or she was _____.

12. Keeping time/travel records requires _____ and _____.

Short Answer

Briefly answer the following questions in the spaces provided.

1. Name three different types of home care providers.

    a. _____

    b. _____

    c. _____

2. List four advantages to working for a home health agency.

    a. _____

    b. _____

    c. _____

    d. _____

3. What are five time and cost values to record?

    a. _____

    b. _____

    c. _____

    d. _____

    e. _____

4. What are five ways to avoid liability when providing home care?

    a. _____

    b. _____

    c. _____

    d. _____

    e. _____

5. What are four types of activities that should be included in the client care record?

    a. _____

    b. _____

    c. _____

    d. _____

Matching

Match the activity or responsibility with the proper home health team member.

Activity/Responsibility   **Health Care Team**

1. _____ May or may not be supportive of client   a. client

2. _____ Writes orders and acts as a consultant and guide   b. family

3. _____ Provides direct client care   c. nursing assistant

4. _____ Person in need of care   d. supervising nurse

5. _____ May act as alternate caregivers   e. physician

6. _____ Provides for client's safety and comfort

7. _____ Makes observations about care that was given

8. _____ Teaches and supervises nursing assistants

9. _____ Requires skilled services

10. _____ Plans care

11. _____ May require assistance with ADLs

12. _____ Completes periodic client assessments

13. _____ Documents observations and care that was given

14. _____ May live in the client's home

Computations

Compute the time spent in each case. (Write the 24-hour time designation for each arrival and departure time in the space provided.)

Arrival Time	Departure Time	Time Spent
1. 8:15 AM _____	8:50 AM _____	_____
2. 10:05 AM _____	11:15 AM _____	_____
3. 11:20 AM _____	1:05 PM _____	_____
4. 2:10 PM _____	3:15 PM _____	_____
5. 3:45 PM _____	4:30 PM _____	_____

Clinical Situations

Briefly describe what the nursing assistant should do in the following home care settings.

1. Mary Johnson, who is 78 years of age, has diabetes mellitus. She requires a bed bath, change of linens, and a blood glucose level check. Your arrival time is 8:20 AM and you leave the client's home at 10:05. Your odometer read 42,738 miles when you left the agency and 42,743 miles when you arrived at the client's home. Compute the time spent with the client and the mileage from the agency to the client's home.

_____

_____

2. Mr. Alleandra is 58 and has a diagnosis of terminal cancer of the bone. Your assignment is to spend an entire evening shift with him. In addition to feeding the client and meeting his comfort needs, Mr. Alleandra is lonely and would like you to keep him company. He likes to play cards and dominoes and to watch TV. Describe your actions.

_____

_____

3. Mrs. Parks has congestive heart failure and tires so easily that she has difficulty carrying out her daily living activities. You are assigned to assist her for an entire shift. The family wants you to wash the floor and windows, vacuum, and do the laundry. These activities are not part of the nursing assistant's job description. Describe your actions.

_____

_____

RELATING TO THE NURSING PROCESS

Write the step of the nursing process that is related to the nursing assistant action.

Nursing Assistant Action	Nursing Process Step
1. The nursing assistant performs only skills she has been taught when providing home care.	_____
2. The nursing assistant and the supervisor discuss the exact care to be given to the homebound client.	_____
3. The nursing assistant keeps careful records of the length of time spent on specific activities when in the client's home.	_____

DEVELOPING GREATER INSIGHT

1. You are assigned to work the night shift in Mrs. Lawrence's home. The client sleeps most of the night but must be awakened to take her medication at 12 midnight and 4:00 AM. Think about what activities you might engage in while the client sleeps.

2. Discuss with classmates the reasons why clients might prefer to have home care rather than remain in a long-term care facility.

3. Invite a nursing assistant who works in home care to share his or her experiences with you.

The Nursing Assistant in Home Care

OBJECTIVES

After completing this unit, you will be able to:

- Spell and define terms.
- Summarize the four levels of hospice care.
- Define core values and explain why they are important.
- Describe the characteristics that are especially important to the nursing assistant who provides home care.
- List at least 10 methods of protecting your personal safety when working as a home care nursing assistant in the community.
- Describe the duties of the nursing assistant who works in the home setting.
- Describe appropriate circumstances for assisting clients with medications and list the "Six Rights" of medication administration.
- Describe the duties of the homemaker assistant.
- Describe methods of food preparation.
- Carry out home care activities needed to maintain a safe and clean environment.

UNIT SUMMARY

There is an increasing trend to provide home health care to housebound, recuperating, and chronically ill clients. The nursing assistant who provides this care may also carry out housekeeping activities.

Home health care consists of:

- Maintaining a safe, comfortable environment for the client.
- Managing infection control.

- Carrying out proper nursing techniques under the supervision of the nurse case manager.

The home health assistant occupies the positions of a:

- Member of the home health care team.
- Guest in the client's home.
- Provider of direct health care and household assistance.

242

NURSING ASSISTANT ALERT

Action	Benefit
Adapt procedures to the home setting following accepted techniques and safety standards.	Ensures that the same standard of care will be given in all health care settings.
Carry out housekeeping duties diligently.	Secures a clean and safe environment for the client.
Be alert to unsafe conditions in the home, and correct or report them.	Prevents injury to client, caregiver, and others.
Adapt procedures to equipment found in the home whenever possible.	Contributes to cost containment.

ACTIVITIES

Vocabulary Exercise

Find the following words in the puzzle and circle them.

y	i	r	t	n	a	t	s	i	s	s	a	l
i	t	n	r	e	i	r	r	a	b	m	e	e
n	o	e	t	g	r	c	z	j	a	v	s	i
f	r	j	f	e	a	g	f	e	a	r	h	s
e	g	u	b	a	r	b	t	r	u	n	t	e
c	a	z	x	u	s	m	t	n	c	a	t	i
t	n	i	a	l	m	/	i	t	y	q	m	l
i	i	r	l	a	e	t	h	t	o	t	d	p
o	z	b	p	m	n	d	z	e	t	q	p	p
u	e	a	i	e	d	d	x	q	e	e	l	u
s	q	t	i	c	j	z	s	w	v	d	n	s
q	k	l	a	l	c	o	h	o	l	m	i	t
s	c	h	o	m	e	m	a	k	e	r	j	a

1. aide

2. alcohol

3. assistant

4. bag

5. barrier

6. client

7. homemaker

8. infectious

9. intermittent

10. map

11. nurse

12. organize

13. safety

14. supplies

15. team

16. time/travel

Completion

Complete the following statements in the spaces provided.

1. The nursing assistant contributes to the planning step of the nursing process by actively participating in _____.

2. The client should, if able, make decisions about food _____.

3. The client's bathroom should be cleaned _____.

4. Before _____ the client's appliances, seek _____ from a family member.

5. Be sure to _____ the _____ off before hanging laundered clothes outside.

6. Before storing clothes that have been laundered, check for needed _____.

7. Drip-dry fabrics should be washed _____ so they can be hung and folded.

8. The primary role of the home health assistant is to _____.

9. The major responsibility of the homemaker assistant is to provide _____.

10. In some cases, the nursing assistant who provides health care may be asked to carry out _____ chores.

11. Because home health assistants handle money, they must be _____ people.

12. The home health care assistant's activities are planned around the _____.

13. To save costs, _____ enema equipment may be substituted for disposable enema equipment.

14. Statements by the client that reflect neglect or abuse should be _____.

15. Chemicals such as household cleaning supplies and insecticides should be kept locked up when the client is _____.

16. Dust, dirty dishes, and improper care of foods contribute to the spread of _____.

Short Answer

Briefly answer the following questions in the spaces provided.

1. What are three areas to report that support the assessment process?

   a. _____

   b. _____

   c. _____

2. What are two ways to support the implementation portion of the nursing process?

   a. _____

   b. _____

3. What are two ways to promote the evaluation part of the nursing process?

   a. _____

   b. _____

4. What are three household duties the nursing assistant frequently performs?

   a. _____

   b. _____

   c. _____

5. What are three household cleaning duties not included in the nursing assistant's responsibilities?

   a. _____

   b. _____

   c. _____

6. What are four kinds of telephone numbers to be kept close to the phone during home care?

   a. _____

   b. _____

   c. _____

   d. _____

7. What action should the nursing assistant take when cleaning laundry soiled by blood?

   _____

8. What are 10 ways of maintaining your personal safety when working in home care?

   a. _____

   b. _____

   c. _____

   d. _____

   e. _____

   f. _____

   g. _____

   h. _____

   i. _____

   j. _____

True/False

Mark the following true or false by circling T or F.

1. T   F   Household duties may be part of the home nursing assistant's responsibilities.

2. T   F   Caring for food properly is part of your responsibility.

3. T   F   It is all right to leave dirty dishes in the sink after the client eats.

4. T   F   Cleaning the client's bathroom and kitchen are part of the nursing assistant's responsibilities.

5. T   F   Fresh fruits that are to be used right away should be stored in the refrigerator.

6. T   F   Dried and canned foods should be stored in the refrigerator.

7. T   F   Dairy products need not be refrigerated until use.

8. T   F   Frozen foods may safely be thawed in the kitchen sink until use.

9. T   F   Dirty dishes left to accumulate will contribute to infection.

10. T   F   Loose scatter rugs are safe to use in the home if the client knows where they are placed.

11. T   F   Electrical outlets that have multiple cords plugged in could cause fires.

12. T   F   Hospice is a philosophy of care that may be given in many locations.

13. T   F   Short-term respite care is available for persons receiving hospice services.

14. T   F   The home care agency is responsible for assessing each client's core values.

15. T   F   The home care nursing assistant is permitted to administer oral medications.

16. T   F   Document the reason and response when the client takes a PRN (as needed) medication.

Matching

Match the words on the right with the statements on the left.

1. _____ Transferring heat by using steam instead of water.   a. Grilling

2. _____ Cooking rapidly in a bubbling liquid.   b. Tossing

3. _____ Dry method of cooking in which oven temperature is determined by sugar content.   c. Pan frying

4. _____ Quick, dry, and very hot method of cooking over a source of constant, direct radiant heat.   d. Boiling

5. _____ Cooking food under a source of direct radiant heat.   e. Simmering

6. _____ Moist-heat, slow cooking method of roasting in which liquid is added to the meat.   f. Steaming

7. _____ Cooking food on stove covered by half with oil.   g. Braising

8. _____ Mixing or shaking small food items.   h. Baking

9. _____ Slow, moist-heat method of cooking food in liquid to break down connective tissue in tough cuts of meat and fiber in some vegetables.   i. Broiling

10. _____ Gently cooking a delicate product in a flavored liquid.   j. Poaching

Clinical Situations

Briefly describe what the nursing assistant could do to address the following situations in the home setting.

1. The bed is not flexible and the client needs to be in a semi-Fowler's position.

   _____

2. The client has sprained an ankle and there is no ice bag to apply cold.

   _____

3. The client needs to remain in bed and likes to do puzzles to pass the time.

   _____

4. The client is very heavy and there is no trapeze to help with lifting and moving.

   _____

5. You must give a bed bath and there is no bath blanket.

   _____

6. The client must remain in bed, so all care must be given on a regular-height twin bed.

   _____

7. The client is a child who, though in traction, has many toys, crayons, and books scattered over the bed.

   _____

8. You need a place to put soiled laundry as you give care.

   _____

9. The client occasionally needs an enema, and disposable enema equipment is too expensive.

   _____

10. The client has an upper respiratory infection, and you must safely dispose of soiled tissues.

    _____

11. You are visiting Mrs. Morrison regularly as part of your assignment. This morning you notice a bruise on her arm, and she tells you that she and her daughter, who lives with her, quarreled last evening. What action should you take?

    _____

    _____

    _____

12. Mary Schroeder is 91 years old and is very frail. She has been diagnosed with emphysema, CHF, and diabetes. She is being cared for by her sister, who is 93 years old. You are assigned to provide personal hygiene care three mornings each week. Ms. Schroeder is in a regular bed that is low to the floor and cannot have its position changed. The client is incontinent. You must adapt her low-income environment to provide proper care.

    _____

    _____

    _____

RELATING TO THE NURSING PROCESS

Write the step of the nursing process that is related to the nursing assistant action.

Nursing Assistant Action   **Nursing Process Step**

1. The nursing assistant reports to her supervisor about improvement in the homebound client's appetite.

   _____

2. The nursing assistant reports that the client receiving home care is now able to function independently.

   _____

3. The nursing assistant informs the supervisor that stress between the client and his daughter about the client's planned activities is interfering with the client's recovery.

   _____

DEVELOPING GREATER INSIGHT

1. Think back to a time when you were under extreme stress. Did you strike out physically or verbally and then were sorry afterward?

2. Make out a shopping list for meals for one day for two people who are on unrestricted diets but limited income. Look through newspapers for coupons and sales that could save money.

3. Look carefully around your own home and try to identify safety factors that could be changed if health care were needed.

Subacute Care

OBJECTIVES

After completing this unit, you will be able to:

- Spell and define terms.
- Describe the purpose of subacute care.
- Explain the differences between acute care, subacute care, and long-term care.
- Describe special procedures provided in the subacute care unit.
- Describe the responsibilities of the nursing assistant when caring for patients receiving subacute care.
- Define sterile technique and explain why it is used.
- List the guidelines for sterile procedures.
- Describe the purpose of a sterile field, and demonstrate how to establish a sterile field.
- Explain when to use sterile gloves, and describe how to use them without contamination.
- Describe the care of surgical drains.
- Describe continuous sutures, interrupted sutures, and staples.
- Demonstrate the following procedures:

  Procedure 88 Setting Up a Sterile Field Using a Sterile Drape
  Procedure 89 Adding an Item to a Sterile Field
  Procedure 90 Adding Liquids to a Sterile Field
  Procedure 91 Applying and Removing Sterile Gloves
  Procedure 92 Using Transfer Forceps
  Procedure 93 Applying a Dry Sterile Dressing
  Procedure 94 Discontinuing a Peripheral IV
  Procedure 95 Applying a Dressing Around a Drain
  Procedure 96 Care of a T-Tube or Similar Wound Drain
  Procedure 97 Removing Sutures
  Procedure 98 Removing Staples

UNIT SUMMARY

Nursing assistants who work in subacute care units must have an advanced education and experience caring for the types of patients found in these units. They must be able to support complex therapies while providing basic nursing care.

Nursing assistants must be prepared to give assistance in the care of patients receiving special therapy, such as:

- Chemotherapy
- Rehabilitation
- Central venous catheter
- Intravenous therapy
- Total parenteral nutrition
- Patient-controlled analgesia (PCA); pain management needs
- Continuous medication infusion through an implanted delivery system

- Epidural catheter approach to pain management
- Transcutaneous electrical nerve stimulation (TENS)
- Tracheostomy
- Oxygen therapy
- Radiation
- Sutures and staples
- Wound management, including surgical and chronic wounds and wounds with drains

Nursing assistants must know:

- The purpose of the therapy.
- Important observations to report.
- Special nursing care techniques.

NURSING ASSISTANT ALERT

Action	Benefit
Participate in inservice education classes.	Develops skills needed to meet specific patient needs.
Seek information in textbooks and professional journals about the specific conditions and care of the types of patients in the unit.	Increases understanding of the reasons for and ways special techniques are carried out.
Participate in interdisciplinary team conferences.	Increases understanding of specific patients and their care. Assures that each individual patient will receive optimum care.

ACTIVITIES

Vocabulary Exercise

Match the terms on the right with the definitions on the left.

1. _____ Care and treatment of persons with cancer

2. _____ Drugs given to relieve severe pain

3. _____ Additional bag of fluid added to the main IV line

4. _____ Artificial opening in trachea

5. _____ Subacute care

a. TENS

b. T-tube

c. chemotherapy

d. spasticity

e. Hemovac

6. _____ Sudden, frequent, involuntary muscle contractions that impair function

7. _____ Mild, harmless electrical current that blocks the transmission of pain to the brain

8. _____ Use of drugs to kill cancer cells in the body

9. _____ Closed drainage system that uses a vacuum unit to remove wound drainage

10. _____ Drain used to remove bile and keep the common bile duct open

f. narcotic analgesics

g. oncology

h. piggyback

i. tracheostomy

j. transitional care

Completion

Complete the following statements in the spaces provided. Select the proper terms from the list provided.

approaches	areas	consistency	emotional
goals	hyperalimentation	participate	peripheral
skilled nursing	transitional	3 to 4 weeks	

1. Subacute care is sometimes referred to as _____ care.

2. Subacute care units are usually located in _____ facilities.

3. Most patients remain in a subacute unit for _____.

4. Most subacute care units provide specialized care in one or two primary _____ of practice.

5. Nursing assistants _____ in special inservice education to meet the needs of subacute care patients.

6. Nursing assistants work with other team members to provide for the _____ well-being of the patients.

7. To give proper care, the nursing assistant must know that _____ have been established.

8. The key to successful rehabilitation is _____.

9. IV therapy refers to fluids and medications given directly into a _____ vein.

10. TPN is also called _____.

Short Answer

Briefly answer each question in the spaces provided.

1. What is the purpose of subacute care?

_____

_____

2. Where do patients continue their care after discharge from a subacute care unit?

a. _____

b. _____

c. _____

3. What are five expectations of a nursing assistant who works on a subacute care unit?

   a. _____

   b. _____

   c. _____

   d. _____

   e. _____

4. Name three types of patients who may require intensive rehabilitation.

   a. _____

   b. _____

   c. _____

5. What are two reasons IV therapy is administered with a central venous catheter?

   a. _____

   b. _____

6. What do the letters PICC stand for?

   _____

7. What are four actions the nursing assistant must not take when caring for a patient with an IV?

   a. _____

   b. _____

   c. _____

   d. _____

8. Explain why sterile technique must be used when caring for a wound drain and state whether standard precautions are or are not necessary.

   _____

   _____

9. What are four important observations to report about a patient who is receiving epidural catheter pain relief?

   a. _____

   b. _____

   c. _____

   d. _____

10. What are four observations that should be reported related to the patient with a tracheostomy?

   a. _____

   b. _____

   c. _____

   d. _____

Completion

Complete the following related to care of the patient receiving an IV.

1. Know the _____ rate.

2. Notify the nurse if the drip chamber is _____.

3. Avoid twisting or pulling _____.

4. Make sure the patient does not _____ on the tubing.

5. Observe the needle insertion site for signs of _____.

6. Make sure all _____ in the tubing are secure.

7. Note signs of moisture that might indicate _____.

8. Report signs of _____, _____, or chest or back pain.

True/False

Mark the following true or false by circling T or F.

1. T F Some patients may feel very uncertain when in a subacute care unit.

2. T F Hyperalimentation allows the bowel to rest.

3. T F Inability to move the legs is normal immediately after a spinal medication pump is implanted.

4. T F Never allow the bag of IV fluid to be lower than the patient's arm.

5. T F The dosage for PCA is controlled by equipment that is preset by the nurse.

6. T F An epidural catheter is implanted under the skin near the elbow to administer a local anesthetic.

7. T F The T-tube will drain 300 mL to 500 mL of blood-tinged bile in the first 24 hours after surgery.

8. T F Tongue piercings are harmless fashion statements.

9. T F TENS is a nondrug method of pain relief.

10. T F Patients with implantable medication pumps must always be moved with a transfer belt.

11. T F Cancer may be treated with surgery, radiation, chemotherapy, or a combination of any of these.

12. T F Patients with tracheostomies should be cautioned about using shaving cream around the stoma.

Clinical Situations

Briefly describe how a nursing assistant should react to the following situations.

1. Mrs. Johns's wound appears red, swollen, and has increased, foul-smelling drainage.

_____

_____

RELATING TO THE NURSING PROCESS

Write the step of the nursing process that is related to the nursing assistant action.

Nursing Assistant Action	Nursing Process Step
1. The nursing assistant reports that her patient, who is receiving chemotherapy by IV, has a reddened area at the site of the needle insertion.	_____
2. The nursing assistant reports that the patient, who has an epidural catheter for pain relief, is complaining of numbness in her right leg.	_____
3. The nursing assistant carefully monitors the patient's vital signs following his return from surgery.	_____

DEVELOPING GREATER INSIGHT

1. Invite a nursing assistant who works in subacute care to discuss his or her experiences with you.

2. Visit a subacute care unit. If possible:

   a. Observe a working assistant.

   b. Identify the types of patients on the unit.

Return to the classroom and discuss your experiences with your classmates and instructor.

Alternative, Complementary, and Integrative Approaches to Patient Care

OBJECTIVES

After completing this unit, you will be able to:

- Spell and define terms.
- Define alternative medicine.
- Differentiate alternative practices from complementary and integrative practices.
- List five categories of alternative and complementary therapies.
- Define holistic care.
- List at least three ways in which the nursing assistant supports patients' spirituality.

UNIT SUMMARY

- Alternatives are options that are used instead of conventional health care. Most alternative strategies involve the use of natural products.

- Complementary medicine is a treatment regimen in which alternative practices are combined with conventional health care.

- Like traditional health care, complementary and alternative medicine (CAM) has risks. A CAM program should always be supervised by a physician or other health care practitioner.

- Many CAM therapies are believed to stimulate the body to heal itself. They may also be used to strengthen weak body systems, and reduce or eliminate the discomfort of some conditions.

- Integrative health care involves using both mainstream medical treatments and CAM therapies to treat the patient.

- Standard medical care focuses on treating single body parts or systems. Most integrative medicine practitioners believe in holistic care. Holistic care considers the whole person, including mind, body, and spirit.

- Many CAM therapies are being used in health care facilities today. Some hospitals have CAM units.

- Spirituality and religion may also be a part of nontraditional health care practices.

255

NURSING ASSISTANT ALERT

Action	Benefit
Learn about the CAM therapies being used by patients in your facility. Follow the plan of care in making observations and reinforcing the nurses' teaching.	Ensures patient safety when using a CAM program.
Observe for and report potential side effects and complications of alternative therapy.	Helps detect complications so that the program can be modified promptly.
Assist the patient with meditation, or practicing religion and spirituality, by providing privacy and enhancing comfort through nursing measures.	Helps the patient to relax and focus. Enhances comfort. Relieves stress, facilitates mind and body rest, promotes healing, and helps reduce pain.
Provide emotional support and respect each patient's beliefs and choices even if you do not agree with them.	Shows respect for each patient as an individual and provides patient-focused care. Enhances self-esteem by giving the patient choices and control.

ACTIVITIES

Vocabulary Exercise

Match the term on the right with the information on the left.

1. _____ Promotes proper nervous system function by using spinal adjustments.

2. _____ Uses tiny, thin needles inserted into the body to correct imbalances.

3. _____ Natural system of medicine that originated in India 2,000 years ago.

4. _____ A method of rubbing on the body to stimulate circulation, promote relaxation, and enhance pain relief.

5. _____ Creates a state of altered consciousness in which the mind is more open to suggestion.

6. _____ Involves exposing patients to special lights, in which ultraviolet rays are blocked.

7. _____ Retraining the mind to control physical problems and stress.

8. _____ Physical and mental activities to channel the body's energy.

9. _____ Stimulation of certain areas in hands and feet to treat illness and reduce stress.

10. _____ Using warm glass jars to create suction over various parts of the body.

11. _____ Burning herbal substances on or near the body.

12. _____ Using the imagination to create images.

a. qigong

b. hypnotherapy

c. visualization

d. Ayurveda

e. chiropractic

f. cupping

g. reflexology

h. light therapy

i. massage therapy

j. moxibustion

k. acupuncture

l. biofeedback

Completion

Complete the following statements in the spaces provided using the words below.

chelation	empowered	guided imagery
herbal therapy	holistic	mind
modalities	osteopathy	physician
privilege	supplements	yoga

1. Complementary and alternative therapies should be used only under _____ supervision.

2. A doctor of _____ combines manipulative therapy with traditional medical treatment.

3. _____ is an alternative practice that employs breath control, postures, and relaxation.

4. Caring for patients during very private moments is a _____.

5. _____ uses medicines made from plants.

6. Practitioners of _____ believe that positive changes can be helped to occur by focusing on and visualizing these changes.

7. _____ are nutritional substances used to make up a deficiency.

8. Using CAM therapy may involve different types of treatments, or _____.

9. Practices that consider the whole person are _____.

10. _____ is an intravenous injection of amino acid to improve blood flow in the legs.

11. One principle of integrative health care is that each individual can be _____ to bring greater wellness and healing into his or her own life.

12. Practitioners of some CAM therapies believe that the _____ has a powerful effect on the body's healing process.

Short Answer

Briefly answer each question in the spaces provided.

1. List five ways in which the nursing assistant can help support the patient's spirituality.

    a. _____

    b. _____

    c. _____

    d. _____

    e. _____

2. Explain why some individuals use CAM therapy.

    _____

    _____

    _____

3. List at least four risks associated with using herbs and nutritional supplements.

   a. _____

   b. _____

   c. _____

   d. _____

4. List the five complementary and alternative medicine categories and give a brief explanation of each.

   a. _____

   b. _____

   c. _____

   d. _____

   e. _____

5. Explain why nursing care is holistic.

   _____

   _____

   _____

True/False

Mark the following true or false by circling T or F.

1. T F When a CAM program is used, the patient is a passive participant.

2. T F Complementary therapies can be used to support and strengthen overall health.

3. T F All individuals using a CAM program will receive identical treatment.

4. T F Anthroposophically Extended Medicine (AEM) treats the whole person and not just the disease or symptoms.

5. T F Ayurveda uses essential oils to stimulate the patient's sense of smell.

6. T F The hands do not touch the body directly during therapeutic touch.

7. T F TCM restores the balance between the body and the elements of earth, fire, water, wood, and metal.

8. T F Acupuncture is painful in certain areas of the body.

9. T F Some vitamins and herbs can be toxic.

10. T F Chiropractic adjustments and osteopathic manipulation are identical treatments.

11. T F Dance therapy focuses on use of the senses and self-expression.

12. T F Color therapy affects the mood and emotions.

13. T F Moxibustion is one form of treatment used in TCM.

Vocabulary Exercise

Complete the word-search puzzle by finding and circling the following words.

```
s o A y q J u e v i t a n r e t l a m g c
c a e o i o s t e o p a t h i c t e n t h
W u d g r n S Z t s O o R s y n d a B h i
a c p e a o g T N W M o b g e i y c n e r
M y i p v s l M s m j r r m t c u n y r o
y g r t i r s o N f e e e a o V C o k a p
p o j X e n u a c h n v t m Y H f i c p r
a l v D r n g y m e o i p n y g d t a e a
r o z p l K g J A m o l t O f X u s b u c
e x K i d j d a n n e R R q s H f u d t t
h e U T E V q o m m m l h l J m h b e i i
t l V e R i i r e o h o N t l Y u i e c c
a f g v g t y n e a r o d j b s V x f l N
m e v o a r t W u U i t m a D o L o o T B
o r n l e a Q P A G M H c e l r i m i z L
r g e g r o N C A D M l B e o i e k b a U
a h a y y o g a D V X w u W l p t y i q X
c m i n t e g r a t i v e z e e a i a e J
i h y p n o t h e r a p y s V z O t e r R
v i s u a l i z a t i o n H v s i g h s p
N a t u r o p a t h i c l X C E L a b y g
```

alternative	complementary	hypnotherapy	movement	Reiki
aromatherapy	cupping	imagery	moxibustion	therapeutic
Ayurveda	electromagnetic	integrative	Naturopathic	visualization
biofeedback	energy	massage	osteopathic	yang
chelation	herbs	meditation	prayer	yin
chiropractic	homeopathy	modalities	qigong	yoga
color			reflexology	

RELATING TO THE NURSING PROCESS

Write the step of the nursing process that is related to the nursing assistant action.

Nursing Assistant Action	Nursing Process Step
1. The nursing assistant checks the care plan to determine how to assist the patient with meditation.	_____
2. The nursing assistant informs the nurse that a patient who is using herbal therapy thinks she may be pregnant.	_____
3. The nursing assistant provides privacy when the patient is praying.	_____
4. The nursing assistant attends a care conference and describes how she calmed the patient when she found the patient crying in her room in the dark.	_____
5. The nursing assistant reports that the patient said the OMT and massage helped relieve her pain.	_____
6. The nursing assistant follows the care plan when the patient returns from her radiation treatment.	_____
7. The nursing assistant reports to the nurse that the patient vomited following her chemotherapy, so she did not take her herbs.	_____

Developing Greater Insight

1. Visit a health food store and get information on the use of herbal products and nutritional supplements. Report your findings to the class.

2. Ask a practitioner of a CAM therapy to speak to the class about the advantages and disadvantages of the treatment.

3. Discuss religion and spirituality with your classmates. How are they alike? How are they different?

Body Systems, Common Disorders, and Related Care Procedures

UNIT **38**

Integumentary System

OBJECTIVES

After completing this unit, you will be able to:

- Spell and define terms.
- Review the location and function of the skin.
- Describe some common skin lesions.
- List three diagnostic tests associated with skin conditions.
- Describe nursing assistant actions relating to care of patients with specific skin conditions.
- Identify persons at risk for the formation of pressure ulcers.
- Describe measures to prevent pressure ulcers.
- Describe the stages of pressure ulcer formation and identify appropriate nursing assistant actions.
- List nursing assistant actions in caring for patients with burns.
- State how skin tears occur and describe prevention measures.
- Describe the guidelines for caring for patients with negative-pressure wound therapy.
- Discuss precautions to use when assisting with a pulsatile lavage treatment.
- Describe the importance of nutrition in healing wounds and burns.

- List the guidelines for cleansing and observing a wound.
- Demonstrate the following procedures:

  Procedure 99   Changing a Clean Dressing and Applying a Bandage

  Procedure 100 Applying a Transparent Film Dressing

  Procedure 101 Applying a Hydrocolloid Dressing

UNIT SUMMARY

- The condition of the skin indicates the general health of the body. The presence of various conditions is revealed through skin:

  ○ Color

  ○ Texture

  ○ Lesions or eruptions

- Pressure ulcers result from pressure on the body that interferes with circulation. Pressure ulcers:

  ○ Are more easily prevented than cured.

  ○ May occur in any patient; some people are at higher risk than others.

  ○ Occur in stages that are recognizable and treatable.

- Burns:

  ○ Are classified according to the depth of tissue damage.

  ○ Require special care, often in burn centers.

- Burn therapy involves:

  ○ Analgesics for pain.

  ○ Infection control.

  ○ Replacement of lost fluids and electrolytes.

  ○ Possible skin grafting to repair injured tissue.

  ○ Position changes and support to prevent contractures and deformities.

NURSING ASSISTANT ALERT

Action	Benefit
Observe and carefully describe and report skin lesions.	Establishes proper data for more accurate evaluation.
Identify those patients at risk for pressure ulcers.	Allows timely nursing interventions.
Provide preventive care.	Prevents painful, costly skin breakdown.
Carry out pressure ulcer care as prescribed.	Limits more extensive damage. Promotes repair.
Apply the principles of standard precautions	Reduces the risk of infection.
Report changes in skin and wounds promptly.	Notifies other team members of a potential need for change in the plan of care.

6. What special care will the nursing assistant emphasize when assisting in the care of a burn patient?

    a. _____

    b. _____

    c. _____

    d. _____

    e. _____

    f. _____

7. List four actions that the nursing assistant should take when caring for a patient with a negative pressure wound therapy system.

    a. _____

    b. _____

    c. _____

    d. _____

8. Why is it important to prevent skin tears?

    a. _____

    b. _____

    c. _____

9. Mr. French is in fair physical condition. He is rather lethargic and is ambulatory with assistance. He has limited movement of his left arm and leg, is continent, and eats poorly. He has an open lesion over his left hip. What is his risk of pressure ulcer development?

    _____

    _____

10. Complete the turning wheel to demonstrate your understanding of the principle of relieving pressure.

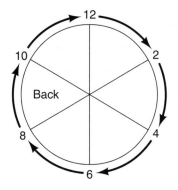

11. List the areas most subject to breakdown when the patient is in the position shown.

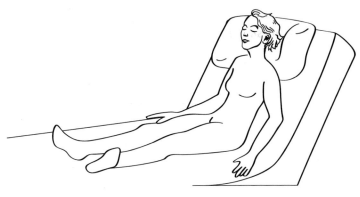

a. _____

b. _____

c. _____

d. _____

e. _____

Clinical Situations

Briefly describe how a nursing assistant should react to the following situations.

1. You burned your finger.

_____

_____

_____

2. You are assigned to give a bed bath and find that the patient has skin lesions.

_____

_____

_____

RELATING TO THE NURSING PROCESS

Write the step of the nursing process that is related to the nursing assistant action.

Nursing Assistant Action   **Nursing Process Step**

1. The nursing assistant charts the presence of excoriation
   on the patient's buttocks.   _____

2. The nursing assistant turns the patient who is in a low-air-loss
   bed every 90 minutes, following the nurse's orders.   _____

3. The nursing assistant reports seeing a pustule on the patient's thigh. _____

4. The nursing assistant makes sure the dependent patient's position is
   changed at least every 2 hours.   _____

5. The nursing assistant uses a turning sheet to move
   dependent patients in bed.   _____

6. The nursing assistant reports an area of irritation around
   the entrance of the nasogastric tube into the patient's nose.   _____

DEVELOPING GREATER INSIGHT

1. What do the following patients have in common: a patient with a nasogastric tube, a patient with an indwelling catheter, and a patient who is able to move independently?

2. Discuss with classmates reasons why changes in the aging integumentary system make the elderly more prone to develop pressure ulcers.

Respiratory System

OBJECTIVES

After completing this unit, you will be able to:

- Spell and define terms.
- Review the location and function of the respiratory organs.
- Describe some common diseases of the respiratory system.
- List five diagnostic tests used to identify respiratory conditions.
- Describe nursing assistant actions related to the care of patients with respiratory conditions.
- Identify patients who are at high risk of poor oxygenation.
- Describe the care of patients with a tracheostomy, laryngectomy, or chest tubes.
- List five safety measures for the use of oxygen therapy.
- Describe the care of patients who have an endotracheal tube and are mechanically ventilated.
- State the purpose of the oral airway and nasal airway, and discuss the care of patients who have airways in place.
- Discuss the use of the incentive spirometer, nebulizer, and CPAP mask.
- Demonstrate the following procedures:

  Procedure 102   Checking Capillary Refill

  Procedure 103   Using a Pulse Oximeter

  Procedure 104   Collecting a Sputum Specimen

UNIT SUMMARY

The organs of respiration function to take in and exchange oxygen and output carbon dioxide. Diseases that affect the respiratory tract make breathing difficult. These conditions include:

- Upper respiratory infections
- Chronic obstructive pulmonary diseases (COPD)
- Malignancies

Patients with many conditions are at high risk of developing hypoxemia, a serious complication. Immobility is a barrier to positive outcomes.

Capillary refill checks and the pulse oximeter are excellent tools for monitoring patients who are at risk of hypoxemia.

The nursing assistant may also care for patients with respiratory conditions who have had surgical intervention:

- Tracheostomy
- Laryngectomy
- Chest tubes

Patients with sleep apnea may wear a continuous positive airway pressure [CPAP] mask, which uses positive pressure to maintain the airway during sleep.

Special techniques that can make breathing easier include:

- Oxygen therapy
- Incentive spirometry
- Positioning
- Mouth care

Special precautions must be taken to avoid transmission of disease. These precautions include handwashing, proper disposal of soiled tissues, and avoidance of coughing and sneezing in the direction of others. Observations that should be reported and documented include:

- Rate and rhythm of respiration.
- Changes in skin color.
- Character and presence of respiratory secretions.
- Cough, including character (for example, amount, color, and odor of sputum, if present).
- Unusual sounds during respiration.
- Abnormal chest movement (or absence of movement).
- Abnormal capillary refill, pulse oximeter values, or rapid pulse.
- Change in mental status.

NURSING ASSISTANT ALERT

Action	Benefit
Use standard precautions when working with patients who have respiratory tract conditions.	Prevents transmission of disease.
Note, report, and document alteration in respiratory patterns or function.	Early interventions can improve ventilation and oxygen exchange.
Be prepared to react quickly and correctly to prevent emergencies involving oxygen use.	Averts possible fire hazards and patient injury.
Follow procedures for sputum specimen collection carefully.	Avoids contamination of specimens. Protects against transmission of infectious materials.
Label and deliver sputum specimens promptly.	Prevents deterioration of specimens that might give false results. Matches the proper findings with the correct patient.

Memorize the normal and abnormal pulse oximeter values.

Identifies potential problems before the patient is symptomatic.

Check the patient's capillary refill.

Shows how well oxygen is getting to body tissues.

ACTIVITIES

Vocabulary Exercise

Complete the puzzle by filling in the missing letters of words found in this unit. Use the definitions to help you discover these words.

1.   __ __ S __ __ __ __   1. Difficult breathing
2.   __ __ P__ __ __ __ __ __ __   2. Bring up material from lungs
3.   __ __ __ __ I __ __ __ __ __   3. Inspiration followed by exhalation
4.   __ R __ __ __ __ __   4. Joins upper respiratory tract to lungs
5.   __ __ __ __ O __ __ __   5. Bluish discoloration of skin due to lack of oxygen
6.   __ __ __ __ M __ __ __ __   6. Serious inflammation of the lungs
7.   __ __ __ E __ __ __   7. Areas of the lungs where oxygen exchange occurs
8.   __ __ T __ __ __   8. Condition caused by narrowing and clogging of the bronchi
9.   __ __ __ __ E __   9. Gas needed for life
10. __ __ R __ __ __   10. Voice box

Definitions

Define the following terms or abbreviations.

1. biopsy

_____

2. sputum

_____

3. URI

_____

4. SOB

_____

5. COPD

_____

6. cannula

_____

7. stoma

_____

8. sleep apnea

_____

Anatomy Review

Using a colored pencil or crayon, fill in the areas on the following figure through which oxygen must flow from the outside to the exchange area. Then name the parts in their proper order.

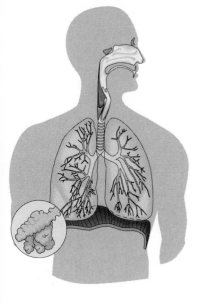

1. _____

2. _____

3. _____

4. _____

5. _____

6. _____

7. _____

Completion

Complete the following statements in the spaces provided.

1. The patient experiencing an asthmatic attack has dyspnea and wheezing because there is increased _____ production, spasm of the _____ tree, and swelling of the _____ lining the respiratory tract.

2. The person with bronchitis has _____ cough.

3. Common allergens include pollen, medications, dust, _____, and _____.

4. Symptoms of a URI include runny nose, watery eyes, and _____.

5. The tiny air sacs forming the lungs are called _____.

6. In emphysema, the alveoli lose some of their _____.

7. Changes in emphysema allow _____ to become trapped in the lungs.

8. The patient with emphysema has the most difficulty in the _____ phase of respiration.

9. It is important for the nursing assistant to know and read the _____ rate of oxygen for each patient.

10. _____ is a condition in which there is insufficient oxygen in the blood.

11. During oxygen administration, the area around the mask should be periodically _____ and _____.

12. The external opening of the tracheostomy is the _____.

13. If a patient has had a _____, the larynx has been removed.

14. Avoid getting _____, _____, _____, or _____ near or in the stoma.

15. _____ are used after chest surgery to drain bloody fluid from the chest.

16. Being unable to _____ is very frightening.

Short Answer

Briefly answer each question in the spaces provided.

1. What four practices should be taught to all patients with upper respiratory infections?

   a. _____

   b. _____

   c. _____

   d. _____

2. What are four observations regarding patients with respiratory disease that must be reported?

   a. _____

   b. _____

   c. _____

   d. _____

3. What are 10 important points about the care of patients with COPD?

   a. _____

   b. _____

   c. _____

   d. _____

   e. _____

   f. _____

   g. _____

   h. _____

   i. _____

   j. _____

4. What precautions must be taken when a patient receives oxygen from a tank?

   a. _____

   b. _____

   c. _____

   d. _____

5. List five conditions that increase the patient's risk of hypoxemia:

   a. _____

   b. _____

   c. _____

   d. _____

   e. _____

6. List eight observations of the patient with chest tubes that require immediate nursing notification.

   a. _____

   b. _____

   c. _____

   d. _____

   e. _____

   f. _____

   g. _____

   h. _____

7. Give three characteristics of the orthopneic position.

   a. _____

   b. _____

   c. _____

8. What are three kinds of breathing exercises that may be ordered for the patient with COPD?

   a. _____

   b. _____

   c. _____

9. What are two other techniques, beside mucolytic medications, used to loosen mucus and clear the air passageways?

   a. _____

   b. _____

10. List four safety precautions specific to the use of liquid oxygen.

   a. _____

   b. _____

   c. _____

   d. _____

Hidden Picture

Carefully study the following picture and identify 7 rules of oxygen safety that have been violated. Write them in the spaces provided. (There are 11.)

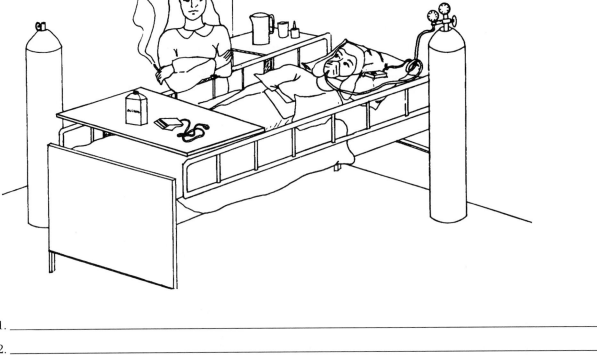

1. _____

2. _____

3. _____

4. _____

5. _____

6. _____

7. _____

Clinical Situations

Briefly describe how a nursing assistant should react to the following situations.

1. You enter a patient's room and find the patient receiving a higher level of oxygen than is ordered.

_____

_____

2. Your patient complains of mouth dryness while receiving oxygen therapy.

_____

_____

3. Your patient who is receiving oxygen therapy wants to shave with an electric razor.

_____

_____

4. You are assigned to collect a sputum specimen for culture and sensitivity. Before collecting a specimen, the patient should _____

   _____

5. Complete the following label, which is attached to a specimen container, using the following information: Mr. James Brown is a patient in room 604. His medical record number is 689473. Dr. Smith has written an order to obtain a sputum specimen for culture and sensitivity testing today.

   Name _____   Room _____

   Date _____   Hospital Number _____

   Doctor _____

   Specimen _____   Examination _____

Matching

Match the words on the right with the statements on the left.

1. _____ Source of water to moisten oxygen

2. _____ Extends from the nostril to the posterior pharynx

3. _____ Tube that provides complete control over the airway

4. _____ Should not be used for liter flows over 5

5. _____ Rigid plastic suction device

6. _____ Device used to manually ventilate a patient

7. _____ Used only for unconscious patients

8. _____ Device used to mechanically ventilate a patient

9. _____ Delivers oxygen through the nose

10. _____ Opening into the body

11. _____ Treatment for sleep apnea

12. _____ Made by cooling oxygen gas

13. _____ Delivers moisture or medication deep into the lungs

14. _____ Prevents atelectasis and pneumonia

a. bag-valve-mask (BVM)

b. continuous positive airway pressure (CPAP)

c. endotracheal tube (ET tube)

d. humidifier

e. incentive spirometer

f. liquid oxygen

g. nasal cannula

h. nasopharyngeal airway

i. nebulizer

j. oropharyngeal airway

k. oxygen concentrator

l. stoma

m. ventilator

n. Yankauer catheter

RELATING TO THE NURSING PROCESS

Write the step of the nursing process that is related to the nursing assistant action.

Nursing Assistant Action   **Nursing Process Step**

1. The nursing assistant makes sure the strap holding a mask
   delivering oxygen is not too tight.   _____

2. The nursing assistant periodically removes an oxygen
   delivery mask and carefully washes and dries the skin underneath it.   _____

3. The nursing assistant reports that the patient's respirations
   have become labored.   _____

4. The nursing assistant keeps the patient's face free
   of any nasal discharge when a nasal airway is in use.   _____

5. The nursing assistant positions pillows behind the patient's
   back to assist his breathing.   _____

6. The nursing assistant helps position the patient so the
   respiratory therapist can give a treatment.   _____

7. The nursing assistant informs the nurse that the oxygen
   flow meter is set lower than the level noted on the care plan.   _____

DEVELOPING GREATER INSIGHT

1. Try wearing an oxygen mask on your face for 20 minutes. Be sure the tubing is open so you have a
   continuous source of air. Describe your feelings when you remove the mask.

2. In the clinical area, practice identifying the number of liters on a flow meter, under supervision.

Circulatory (Cardiovascular) System

OBJECTIVES

After completing this unit, you will be able to:

- Spell and define terms.
- Review the location and functions of the organs of the circulatory system.
- Describe some common disorders of the circulatory system.
- Describe nursing assistant actions related to care of patients with disorders of the circulatory system.
- List five specific diagnostic tests for disorders of the circulatory system.
- State the purpose of the pacemaker and implantable cardioverter defibrillator.

UNIT SUMMARY

The cardiovascular system is the transportation system of the body.

- The heart and blood vessels make up a closed network. This network carries the blood and the products of and for metabolism.

- Diseases that affect the heart or blood vessels often have a related effect on many other parts of the body, especially the respiratory tract.

- Because heart disease is so prevalent, the nursing assistant will likely provide care for many patients with cardiovascular problems.

NURSING ASSISTANT ALERT

Action	Benefit
Do nothing to limit circulation.	Allows patient to make optimum use of cardiovascular function.
Recognize that abnormalities in any part of the cardiovascular system may affect other parts of the body and/or the body as a whole.	Alerts staff to the significance of signs and symptoms in other systems.
Carefully observe, report, and document observations.	Provides a database for appropriate nursing interventions.

ACTIVITIES

Vocabulary Exercise

Unscramble the words introduced in this unit and define them.

1. N A M E A I _____

    _____

2. T O A R A _____

    _____

3. E B L S M U O _____

    _____

4. C E S H I I M A _____

    _____

5. H T M R U B O S _____

    _____

6. P R Y T O H Y E P R H _____

    _____

7. I N G N A A _____

    _____

8. D E U I S R I S _____

    _____

9. T R H M A A E O _____

    _____

10. Y R I D S S A A S C _____

    _____

Anatomy Review

Name the valves located between:

1. The right atrium and the right ventricle _____
2. The left atrium and the left ventricle _____
3. The right ventricle and the pulmonary artery _____
4. The left ventricle and the aorta _____

5. Using colored pencils or crayons, color the venous blood blue and the arterial blood red in the following figure.

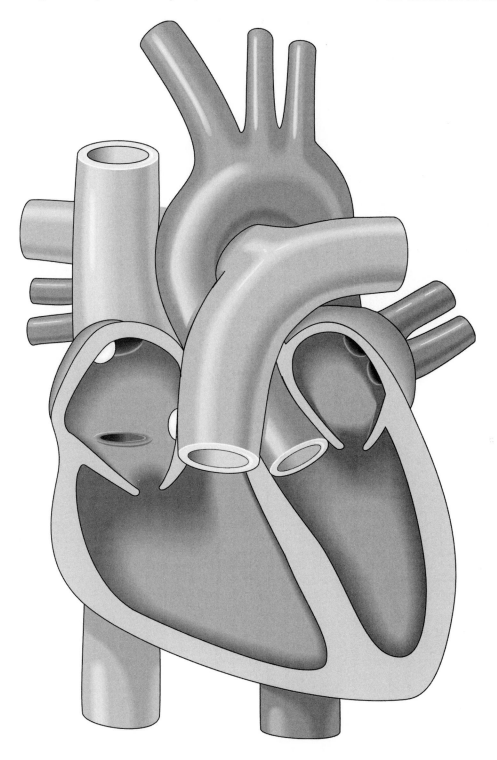

Label the Diagram

Trace the flow of blood from the heart to the lungs, then back to the heart.

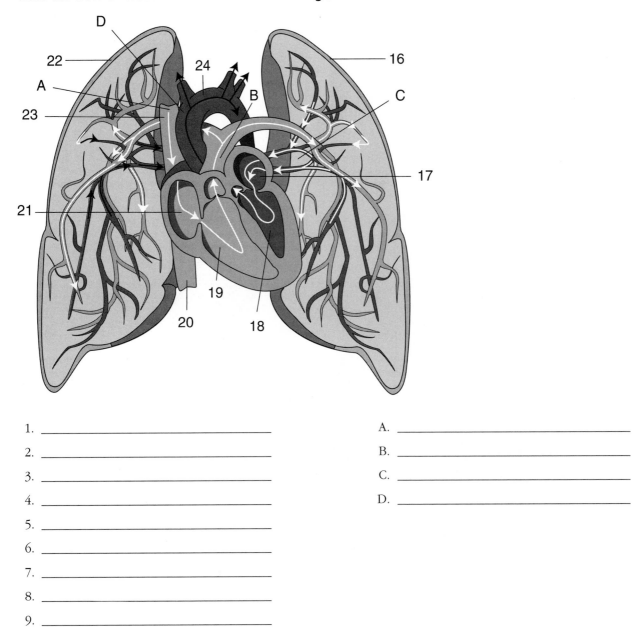

1. _____
2. _____
3. _____
4. _____
5. _____
6. _____
7. _____
8. _____
9. _____

A. _____
B. _____
C. _____
D. _____

Completion

Complete the following statements in the spaces provided.

1. Patients who have long-standing cardiac disease often develop diseases of the _____ system and the _____ system.

2. Blood vessels that serve the outer parts of the body are called _____ blood vessels.

3. Blood abnormalities are referred to as blood _____.

4. Following prescribed exercises carefully can help promote _____ flow and _____ return.

5. The diet of the person who is hypertensive usually limits the amount of _____ intake.

6. Angioplasty is a surgical procedure to _____ blood vessels.

7. Coronary bypass is a surgical procedure that _____ blocked arteries.

8. When the coronary muscles are blocked, the heart tissue becomes _____.

Short Answer

Briefly answer the following questions.

1. List 10 nursing assistant responsibilities in caring for the feet of patients with peripheral vascular disease.

   a. _____

   b. _____

   c. _____

   d. _____

   e. _____

   f. _____

   g. _____

   h. _____

   i. _____

   j. _____

2. Which observations would be reported about patients with circulatory disorders?

   a. _____

   b. _____

   c. _____

   d. _____

   e. _____

3. What six signs and symptoms indicate decreased circulation to an area?

   a. _____

   b. _____

   c. _____

   d. _____

   e. _____

   f. _____

4. To what part of the body do the vessels lead that are most commonly affected by atherosclerosis and the formation of atheromas?

   a. _____

   b. _____

   c. _____

5. What seven conditions predispose a person to the development of atherosclerosis?

   a. _____

   b. _____

   c. _____

   d. _____

   e. _____

   f. _____

   g. _____

6. What four factors are stressed in treatment of the patient with atherosclerosis?

   a. _____

   b. _____

   c. _____

   d. _____

7. What four diagnostic medical terms are used to indicate a coronary heart attack?

   a. _____

   b. _____

   c. _____

   d. _____

8. What three special observations must the nursing assistant note when caring for a patient who is recovering from an MI?

   a. _____

   b. _____

   c. _____

9. What four signs or symptoms might be noted and reported in the patient with CHF?

   a. _____

   b. _____

   c. _____

   d. _____

10. What seven nursing care procedures would the nursing assistant carry out for the patient with CHF?

   a. _____

   b. _____

   c. _____

   d. _____

   e. _____

   f. _____

   g. _____

True/False

Mark the following true or false by circling T or F.

1. T F A rocking bed is used to lull the patient into relaxation.

2. T F The patient with peripheral vascular disease should avoid sitting with the legs crossed.

3. T F The safest way to supply warmth to a patient with peripheral vascular disease is to apply a heating pad.

4. T F People with poor peripheral circulation should avoid smoking.

5. T F In atherosclerosis, blood vessels become widely dilated.

6. T F Severe, crushing chest pain may be a symptom of an MI.

7. T F Heart failure is also known as PVD.

8. T F The anemic patient may require special mouth care.

9. T F The anemic person is pale and may experience exhaustion and dyspnea.

10. T F Sickle cell anemia is due to an inability to absorb vitamin B12.

11. T F The nursing care of the person with leukemia is similar to that given to the person with anemia.

12. T F The patient with a pacemaker must hold a cell phone or cordless phone on the opposite side of the body from the pacemaker.

13. T F Persons with pacemakers should not be in the same room with a microwave oven.

14. T F A pacemaker must be replaced every four years.

15. T F The nursing assistant will be shocked if he or she is touching a patient when an ICD delivers a shock.

16. T F Ventricular dysrhythmias occur in the lower chambers of the heart.

17. T F A stent keeps the arteries open.

18. T F Sickle cell anemia is seen most often in persons of Mediterranean descent.

Clinical Situations

Briefly describe how a nursing assistant should react to the following situations.

1. Your patient, who has angina pectoris, is having an argument with a visitor.

   _____

   _____

2. You are passing out meal trays and find a salt packet on the tray of a patient who has congestive heart failure.

   _____

3. The patient with congestive heart failure has an erratic radial pulse rate of 72.

   _____

4. The patient with congestive heart failure has a fluid intake far in excess of output.

   _____

   _____

5. Your patient who has hypertension suddenly complains of blurred vision and his speech is slurred.

   _____

   _____

RELATING TO THE NURSING PROCESS

Write the step of the nursing process that is related to the nursing assistant action.

Nursing Assistant Action	Nursing Process Step
1. The nursing assistant reports that the resident's legs are pale and cool to the touch.	_____
2. The nursing assistant weighs the patient who has congestive heart failure daily.	_____
3. The nursing assistant completes the bath for the patient who has congestive heart failure, to lessen fatigue.	_____
4. The nursing assistant provides special mouth care for the patient with anemia.	_____
5. The nursing assistant reports that the patient who is anemic tires very easily.	_____

DEVELOPING GREATER INSIGHT

1. Think through reasons why the patient with peripheral vascular disease should wear properly fitting shoes when out of bed.

2. Discuss with classmates the kinds of concerns you might have if you were dependent on a pacemaker.

3. Practice finding and measuring the pulse in each of the following vessels:

   a. temporal

   b. carotid

   c. popliteal

   d. dorsalis pedis

4. Think through why people who cross their legs, sit long hours at work, or have the heavy weight of pregnancy in the abdomen tend to develop varicose veins.

Musculoskeletal System

OBJECTIVES

After completing this unit, you will be able to:

- Spell and define terms.
- Describe the location and functions of the musculoskeletal system.
- Describe some common conditions of the musculoskeletal system.
- Describe nursing assistant actions related to the care of patients with conditions and diseases of the musculoskeletal system.
- List at least seven specific diagnostic tests for musculoskeletal conditions.
- Demonstrate the following procedures:

   Procedure 105   Assisting with Continuous Passive Motion

   Procedure 106   Performing Range-of-Motion Exercises (Passive)

UNIT SUMMARY

- Orthopedic injuries often require long periods of immobilization and rehabilitation.

- Routine range-of-motion exercises must be carried out for all uninjured joints to:
  - Prevent deformities and joint stiffening
  - Promote general circulation
  - Prevent mineral loss from the bones

- Special nursing care for patients with fractures, hip prostheses, joint replacement, and other orthopedic surgery:
  - Ensures proper alignment
  - Prevents pressure areas
  - Avoids skin breakdown

- Continuous passive motion (CPM) therapy is often ordered to reduce the risk of complications following joint replacement and other orthopedic procedures.

- Compartment syndrome is a serious complication of injury and orthopedic surgery. This painful condition occurs when pressure within the muscles builds up, preventing blood and oxygen from reaching muscles and nerves.

- Osteoporosis is a metabolic disorder in which bone mass is lost, causing bones to become porous and spongy and fracture more easily.

- Fibromyalgia is a common chronic pain syndrome for which there is no known cause or cure.

NURSING ASSISTANT ALERT

Action	Benefit
Encourage activity that is consistent with individual patient limitations.	Prevents loss of mobility.
	Helps prevent the development of contractures.
Maintain and promote proper alignment.	Encourages optimum functional ability.
Carry out range-of-motion exercises for patients who are unable to do so themselves.	Maintains mobility and prevents contractures.

ACTIVITIES

Vocabulary Exercise

Each line has four different spellings of a word. Circle the correctly spelled word.

1. barsitis   bursitis   bursites   buresitis
2. cartilage   cartalage   cartilege   catelage
3. comminnuted   cominuted   comminooted   comminuted
4. suppinachon   suppination   supination   suppinasion
5. virtebrae   vertabrae   vertebrae   vertobrae
6. extension   extinsion   extenchon   extention
7. aduction   adducsion   adduchon   adduction
8. dorsiflexion   dorseflexion   dorsiflextion   dorsifection

Anatomy Review

Using colored pencils or crayons, color in the following bones as indicated.

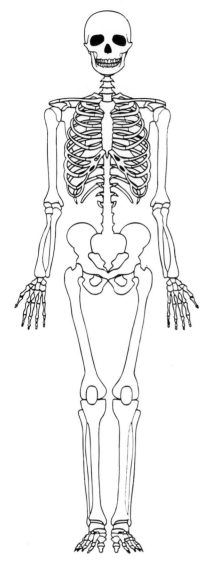

1. femur—red

2. humerus—blue

3. ribs—brown

4. ulna—green

5. radius—red

6. sternum—brown

7. pelvis—blue

8. cranium—green

9. tibia—yellow

Matching

Match the term on the right with the information on the left. Answers may be used more than once.

1. Collapses bone inward; seen only in the vertebrae of the spine

2. Involves only part of the cross-section of bone

3. Breaks completely across the bone

4. Occurs when the fragment from one bone is wedged into another bone

5. Shattering and splintering of the bone into more than three fragments

6. Seen only in fractures of the skull and face; collapses bone fragments inward

7. Runs at an angle across the bone

8. Twists around the bone

9. Fracture in a diseased bone

10. Occurs when a bone fragment is pulled off at the point of ligament or tendon attachment

11. Occurs when only one side of the bone is broken and the other side is bent; common in children

12. Break across the entire cross-section of the bone

13. Improperly aligned

14. Occurs when the skin is intact and not broken

15. Occurs when the skin over the fracture is broken

16. An area containing many blood vessels that bleeds readily when a bone is fractured

a. spiral fracture

b. pathologic fracture

c. depressed fracture

d. avulsion fracture

e. complete fracture

f. oblique fracture

g. greenstick fracture

h. comminuted fracture

i. incomplete fracture

j. displaced

k. transverse fracture

l. closed fracture

m. compound fracture

n. impacted fracture

o. compression fracture

p. vascular

Completion

Complete the statements in the spaces provided.

1. To remain healthy, the musculoskeletal system must be _____

2. Abnormal shortening of muscles is called _____.

3. Moving each toe away from the second toe is called _____.

4. Moving each finger toward the middle finger is called _____.

5. Touching the thumb to the little finger of the same hand is called _____.

6. Rolling the hip in a circular motion toward the midline is called _____.

7. Small fluid-filled sacs found around joints are called _____.

8. Inflammation of a joint is called _____.

9. Any break in the continuity of a bone is a _____.

10. If the broken bone protrudes through the skin, it is called a/an _____ fracture.

11. Traction that uses several weights and lines is called _____ traction.

Short Answer

Briefly answer the following questions.

1. What are four dangers of insufficient exercise?

   a. _____

   b. _____

   c. _____

   d. _____

2. What five special techniques should you use when carrying out ROM exercises?

   a. _____

   b. _____

   c. _____

   d. _____

   e. _____

3. What five techniques are used to treat chronic arthritis?

   a. _____

   b. _____

   c. _____

   d. _____

   e. _____

4. What are five ways to immobilize a fracture?

   a. _____

   b. _____

   c. _____

   d. _____

   e. _____

5. What two special beds are sometimes used when patients have multiple fractures?

   a. _____

   b. _____

6. What eight special nursing care procedures must be given to the patient who is in a fresh plaster leg cast?

   a. _____

   b. _____

   c. _____

   d. _____

   e. _____

   f. _____

   g. _____

   h. _____

7. What are four general factors to keep in mind as care is given to the patient who is in traction?

   a. _____

   b. _____

   c. _____

   d. _____

8. Define the following range-of-motion terms.

   a. extension

   _____

   b. abduction

   _____

   c. rotation: lateral

   _____

   d. eversion

   _____

   e. inversion

   _____

   f. pronation

   _____

   g. radial deviation

   _____

   h. ulnar deviation

   _____

   i. plantar flexion

   _____

   j. dorsiflexion

   _____

9. List two changes that may occur after a cast dries that suggest infection or ulceration under the cast.

   a. _____

   b. _____

10. List six general orders following hip surgery.

   a. _____

   b. _____

   c. _____

   d. _____

   e. _____

   f. _____

11. List four general orders following joint replacement surgery.

    a. _____

    b. _____

    c. _____

    d. _____

12. List six benefits of continuous passive motion therapy.

    a. _____

    b. _____

    c. _____

    d. _____

    e. _____

    f. _____

13. List four contraindications to CPM therapy.

    a. _____

    b. _____

    c. _____

    d. _____

14. List four observations that would cause you to stop the CPM device and promptly report to the nurse.

    a. _____

    b. _____

    c. _____

    d. _____

15. List 10 signs or symptoms of compartment syndrome.

    a. _____

    b. _____

    c. _____

    d. _____

    e. _____

    f. _____

    g. _____

    h. _____

    i. _____

    j. _____

16. Identify the fractures by writing the proper names in the spaces provided.

   a. _____

   A

   c. _____

   C

   b. _____

   B

   d. _____

   D

17. Contrast two forms of chronic arthritis.

Form	Tissue Affected	Possible Cause	Age Affected
Rheumatoid arthritis	_____ _____	_____ _____	_____ _____
Osteoarthritis	_____ _____	_____ _____	_____ _____

18. Figures A and B represent two patients who each have a new right hip prosthesis. Identify the incorrect behavior being demonstrated.

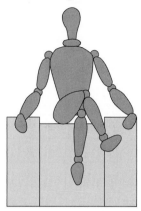

A. _____

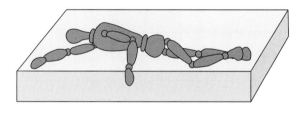

B. _____

Clinical Situations

Briefly describe how a nursing assistant should react to the following situations.

1. The toes of your patient in a leg cast felt cold and looked bluish. _____

_____

_____

2. Your patient has fibromyalgia. Despite receiving pain medication an hour ago, she is crying and says she has severe pain.

_____

_____

_____

3. You find Mr. Lossero, an 82-year-old confused patient, on the floor. His right leg is shortened and externally rotated.

_____

_____

_____

4. Mrs. Huynh has a short leg cast, which is dry. She has an order to take a shower.

   _____

   _____

   _____

5. Your patient has an order for CPM therapy. You take her vital signs and discover that she has a fever and pulse of 104.

   _____

   _____

   _____

6. Your patient has a fractured tibia and fractured radius. Both extremities are casted in plaster casts. You enter the room and the patient tells you that the pain in her tibia is agonizing—even worse than it was when she fell and broke it.

   _____

   _____

   _____

7. Your patient complained of discomfort during range-of-motion exercises.

   _____

   _____

8. The patient has had a lower leg amputated below the knee. You must position the extremity.

   _____

   _____

RELATING TO THE NURSING PROCESS

Write the step of the nursing process that is related to the nursing assistant action.

Nursing Assistant Action	Nursing Process Step
1. The nursing assistant handles the wet cast with open palms.	_____
2. The nursing assistant supports each joint above and below while exercising that joint.	_____
3. The nursing assistant stops carrying out range of motion and reports to the nurse when the patient complains of pain.	_____
4. The nursing assistant carries out each ROM exercise five times.	_____
5. The nursing assistant reports the patient's feelings of numbness in the toes of the newly casted leg.	_____
6. The nursing assistant helps support the patient in a spica cast while another assistant changes the linen.	_____
7. The nursing assistant is very careful not to disturb the weights while caring for the patient with skeletal traction.	_____
8. The nursing assistant asks the nursing supervisor to review the traction lines on the skeletal traction before she begins to give care.	_____

DEVELOPING GREATER INSIGHT

1. Stand in front of a full-length mirror. Be sure you have something to hang onto for support. Raise one leg, bending it at the knee, and pretend that you have had an amputation. How do you feel about your body image now?

2. Wrap one leg in an Ace bandage so you will keep your knee straight, simulating a cast. Try to ambulate safely using crutches. Identify difficulties that a patient in a similar situation might have.

3. Put your dominant arm in a sling and try to carry out your activities of daily living. Did you feel frustrated by the experience?

4. Working in pairs, take turns being patient and nursing assistant and practice passive ROM exercises.

Endocrine System

OBJECTIVES

After completing this unit, you will be able to:

- Spell and define terms.
- Review the location and functions of the endocrine system.
- List five specific diagnostic tests associated with conditions of the endocrine system.
- Describe some common diseases of the endocrine system.
- Recognize the signs and symptoms of hypoglycemia and hyperglycemia.
- Describe nursing assistant actions related to the care of patients with disorders of the endocrine system.
- Perform blood tests for glucose levels if facility policy permits.
- Perform the following procedure:

    Procedure 107   Obtaining a Fingerstick Blood Sugar

UNIT SUMMARY

Endocrine glands:

- Secrete hormones that influence body activities.
- Are subject to disease and malfunction.

Common conditions of the endocrine system are those involving:

- The thyroid gland. These are hyperthyroidism or hypothyroidism.
- The pancreas. A major condition is diabetes mellitus.

Diabetes mellitus:

- Affects many people.

- May be treated with a balance of:
  - Diet
  - Exercise
  - Hypoglycemic drugs or insulin
- Requires conscientious nursing care to avoid serious complications.
- Requires understanding by the patient of the need to follow the therapeutic program.

NURSING ASSISTANT ALERT

Action	Benefit
Know the signs and symptoms of impending diabetic coma and insulin shock and report them at once.	Early intervention can prevent serious complications.
Give special attention to the diabetic's feet and dietary intake.	Contributes to foot health and proper blood sugar levels.
Follow orders faithfully and report response.	Helps stabilize hormonal imbalances.

ACTIVITIES

Vocabulary Exercise

Complete the puzzle by filling in the missing letters of words found in this unit. Use the definitions to help you discover these words.

1. _ _ _ _ _ _ E
2. _ _ _ _ _ N _
3. _ _ _ _ _ D _ _ _
4. _ _ _ _ O _ _ _ _
5. _ _ _ C _ _ _ _ _ _
6. _ _ R _ _ _ _ _
7. _ _ _ I _ _
8. _ _ _ N _ _ _
9. _ _ E _ _

1. blood sugar
2. endocrine secretion
3. being diseased
4. produced by thyroid gland
5. sugar in the urine
6. glands located on top of kidneys
7. needed for production of thyroxine
8. organs that secrete body fluids
9. male reproductive cell

Definitions

Define the following terms or abbreviations in the spaces provided.

1. BMR

2. hypersecretion

3. hypertrophy

4. mortality rate

5. polydipsia

_____

6. tetany

_____

Anatomy Review

Using colored pencils, color the glands as indicated.

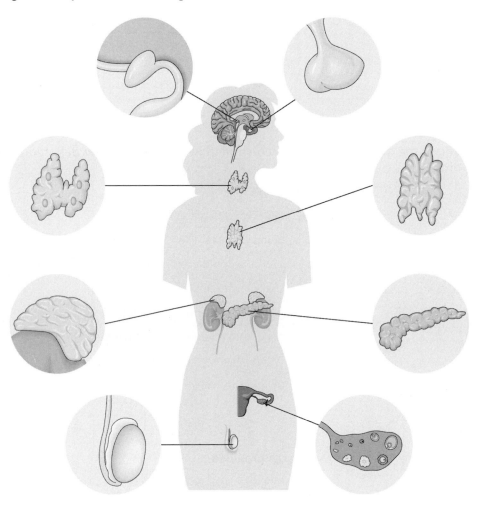

1. ovaries—red

2. thyroid—green

3. pituitary—blue

4. parathyroids—black

5. adrenals—brown

6. pancreas—red

7. pineal body—green

8. testes—yellow

Completion

Complete the following statements in the spaces provided.

1. The role of glands in the body is to secrete _____.

2. The chemicals secreted by glands _____ body activities and growth.

3. A major contribution the nursing assistant can make to the care of a patient with hyperthyroidism is to keep the room _____ and be patient and calm.

4. The treatment for hyperthyroidism is to _____ the level of thyroxine production.

5. Hypothyroidism can occur even when the thyroid gland _____.

6. The role of parathormone is to regulate the electrolyte levels of _____ and
_____.

7. One of the severe effects of inadequate levels of parathormone is acute muscle spasm called
_____.

8. Hypersecretion of adrenal cortical hormones causes a disease syndrome called

_____.

9. The patient with Addison's disease becomes dehydrated and has a low tolerance to

_____.

10. The diabetic exchange system was formulated by a committee with representatives from the
_____ and the diabetes branch of the _____.

11. Measurement of foods in the exchange system is based on standard _____ measurements.

12. Beside diet and insulin, another important part of diabetic therapy is _____.

13. Two medications given for diabetes mellitus are insulin and _____ drugs.

14. The patient with diabetes has a sweet, fruity odor to the breath, so you might suspect

_____.

15. The patient with diabetes is feeling excited, nervous, and hungry, so you might suspect

_____.

16. All urine being tested for acetone must be _____ voided.

17. Daily foot care for the diabetic includes washing, drying, and _____ the feet.

18. Toenails of the diabetic should be cut only by a _____.

19. Diabetic patients should never be permitted to go _____.

20. The radioactive iodine uptake test is performed to check _____.

21. Special care must be taken of the _____ of the patient with diabetes.

Short Answer

Briefly answer the following questions.

1. How might the person with hyperthyroidism look and behave?

_____

_____

2. Your patient has just returned from surgery following a partial thyroidectomy. What should you check for and report?

   a. _____

   b. _____

   c. _____

   d. _____

   e. _____

   f. _____

3. What five factors seem to play a role in the incidence of diabetes mellitus?

   a. _____

   b. _____

   c. _____

   d. _____

   e. _____

4. What complications are common to the patient who suffers uncontrolled diabetes mellitus for many years?

   a. _____

   b. _____

   c. _____

   d. _____

   e. _____

   f. _____

   g. _____

   h. _____

5. What role does diet play in care of the diabetic patient?

   _____

6. What six factors can contribute to a hyperglycemic state?

   a. _____

   b. _____

   c. _____

   d. _____

   e. _____

   f. _____

7. What eight factors can contribute to a hypoglycemic state?

   a. _____

   b. _____

   c. _____

   d. _____

   e. _____

   f. _____

   g. _____

   h. _____

8. What are the nine nursing assistant responsibilities in caring for the patient with insulin-dependent diabetes mellitus?

   a. _____

   b. _____

   c. _____

   d. _____

   e. _____

   f. _____

   g. _____

   h. _____

   i. _____

9. What are the typical signs and symptoms associated with IDDM?

   a. _____

   b. _____

   c. _____

   d. _____

10. What do the abbreviations stand for?

   a. IDDM _____

   b. NIDDM _____

11. What daily care should be given to the feet of the patient with diabetes?

   a. _____

   b. _____

   c. _____

   d. _____

   e. _____

   f. _____

12. Compare the signs and symptoms of diabetic coma and insulin shock.

	Diabetic Coma	**Insulin Shock**
Respirations	_____	_____
Pulse	_____	_____
Skin	_____	_____

Clinical Situations

Briefly describe how a nursing assistant should react to the following situations.

1. Your patient is to have a BMR at 8:00 AM.

   _____

   _____

2. Your older obese patient complains of constant fatigue and burning on urination. She has a bruise on her leg that is healing poorly.

   _____

   _____

3. Your postoperative thyroidectomy patient has increasing difficulty speaking.

   _____

   _____

4. Your postoperative thyroidectomy patient has moved down in the bed so that his neck is hyperextended.

   _____

   _____

RELATING TO THE NURSING PROCESS

Write the step of the nursing process that is related to the nursing assistant action.

Nursing Assistant Action	Nursing Process Step
1. The nursing assistant reports that her patient, a diabetic, has diarrhea.	_____
2. The nursing assistant makes sure the room of the patient with hyperthyroidism is kept cool and quiet.	_____
3. The nursing assistant documents the amount of fluid that the patient with diabetes is consuming.	_____
4. The nursing assistant reports that the patient with diabetes has pale, moist skin and seems nervous.	_____
5. The nursing assistant tests the patient's urine for acetone using the Ketostix strip test.	_____
6. The nursing assistant carefully washes and inspects the feet of the patient with diabetes daily.	_____

DEVELOPING GREATER INSIGHT

1. Make a list of ways your life would change if you were diagnosed with diabetes mellitus type 2. Share your list with the class.

2. Test your own urine for acetone using a Ketostix strip tape.

Nervous System

OBJECTIVES

After completing this unit, you will be able to:

- Spell and define terms.
- State the location and functions of the organs of the nervous system.
- List five diagnostic tests used to determine conditions of the nervous system.
- Describe 15 common conditions of the nervous system.
- Describe nursing assistant actions related to the care of patients with conditions of the nervous system.
- Explain the proper care, handling, and insertion of an artificial eye.
- Explain the proper care, handling, and insertion of a hearing aid.
- Demonstrate the following procedures:

  Procedure 108   Caring for the Eye Socket and Artificial Eye

  Procedure 109   Applying Warm or Cool Eye Compresses

UNIT SUMMARY

The nursing assistant assists the professional nurse in the care of patients with neurological conditions. Although the nurse is responsible for neurological assessment and intervention, an alert nursing assistant can make valuable observations.

- If the nursing assistant notes changes in level of consciousness, response, or behavior, he reports the changes accurately and promptly.
- The nursing assistant supplies comfort and support during the critical care period.

- Under supervision, the nursing assistant provides specific care for patients who have the following conditions:

  ○ CVAs

  ○ Seizures

  ○ Head injuries

  ○ Spinal cord injuries

  ○ Diseases of or trauma to the eyes and ears

- ○ Meningitis

- ○ Parkinson's disease

- ○ Multiple sclerosis

- ○ Post-polio syndrome (PPS)

- ○ Amyotrophic lateral sclerosis (ALS)

- ○ Huntington's disease (HD)

Diseases and injuries of the nervous system often require a long recovery period. During the period of convalescence, the nursing assistant plays an important role. Patience, empathy, and skill are needed in full measure to assist these patients in their recovery.

The nursing assistant must understand the cause and identify signs and symptoms of autonomic dysreflexia. This condition is a potentially life-threatening complication of spinal cord injury that occurs in patients with injuries above the mid-thoracic area.

NURSING ASSISTANT ALERT

Action	Benefit
Document observations and care accurately.	Provides a database for correct nursing evaluations and interventions.
Patiently use a variety of communication skills.	Lessens patient frustration. Improves accuracy in sending and receiving messages.
Be consistent in care and use established routines.	Requires fewer stressful adjustments for the patient.

ACTIVITIES

Vocabulary Exercise

Complete the crossword puzzle by using the definitions provided.

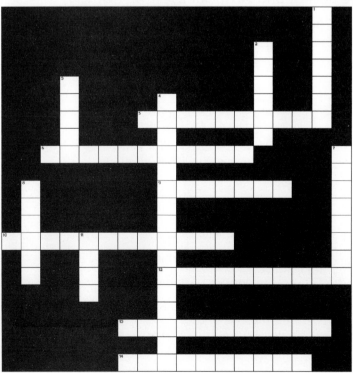

Across

5 Paralysis on one side of the body

6 Weakness on one side of the body, usually caused by a stroke

9 Involuntary and rhythmic shaking movements in the muscles of parts of the body, usually the hands, feet, jaw, tongue, and head

10 Within the skull

12 Paralysis affecting one limb only

13 Paralysis of the trunk (usually below the neck), both arms, and both legs

14 Paralysis of the trunk (usually below the waist) and both legs

Down

1 Organ of hearing in the inner ear

2 Abnormal, involuntary, jerking movements

3 An enclosed, cable-like bundle of nerve fibers (axons and dendrites); part of the peripheral nervous system responsible for sending and receiving messages

4 Specialized chemical messenger that sends a message from one nerve cell to another; the chemical needed for nerve transmission

7 Paralysis affecting the same region on both sides of the body

8 Part of the eye in front of the lens

11 Portion of the neuron that carries the impulse of the cell

Definitions

Define the following terms or abbreviations in the spaces provided.

1. akinesia

_____

2. ossicles

_____

3. aphasia

_____

4. meninges

_____

5. tremors

_____

6. paralysis

_____

7. Lhermitte's sign

_____

8. tetraplegia

_____

9. nystagmus

_____

10. convulsion

_____

Anatomy Review

Using colored pencils, markers, or crayons, color the functional areas of the brain as indicated.

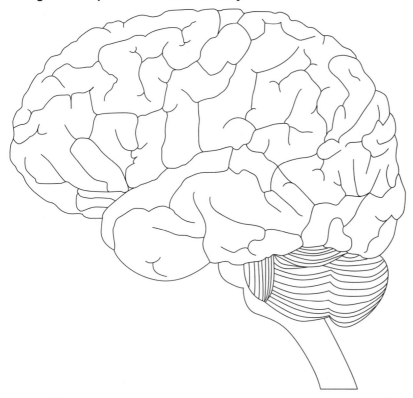

1. movement—red

2. hearing—yellow

3. pain and other sensations—green

4. seeing—brown

5. speech and language—blue

6. spinal cord—black

Completion

Complete the following statements in the spaces provided.

1. The pressure of tissue and fluid within the skull is called _____ pressure.

2. Other names for stroke are _____ or cerebrovascular accident.

3. The symptoms of a stroke depend on the area of _____ that is affected.

4. Left-brain damage often results in loss of _____.

5. Poststroke patients have a high level of _____.

6. TIAs are sometimes called _____.

7. The incidence of macular degeneration increases with _____.

8. Following cataract surgery, the patient should avoid _____.

9. Following cataract surgery, it is especially important to report _____ in the operative eye.

10. Otitis media is an infection of the _____ and may result in _____ of the ossicles, leading to deafness.

11. It is important not to let a hearing aid get _____.

12. Patients with post-polio syndrome are very sensitive to _____, particularly in the feet and legs.

13. Patients with post-polio syndrome need close _____ after surgery because they commonly experience complications.

14. Amyotrophic lateral sclerosis is a progressive neuromuscular disease that causes muscle weakness and _____.

15. _____ acuity is intact in patients with amyotrophic lateral sclerosis.

16. The most common cause of autonomic dysreflexia is _____.

17. Glaucoma is a condition in which the pressure is _____ within the eye.

Short Answer

Briefly answer the following questions.

1. What are six signs that the intracranial pressure is rising in a patient with a head injury?

   a. _____

   b. _____

   c. _____

   d. _____

   e. _____

   f. _____

2. In what four ways can the nursing assistant help the aphasic patient communicate?

   a. _____

   b. _____

   c. _____

   d. _____

3. What eight nursing care measures must be carried out when caring for the patient in the acute phase of a cerebrovascular accident?

   a. _____

   b. _____

   c. _____

   d. _____

   e. _____

   f. _____

   g. _____

   h. _____

4. List eight signs and symptoms of post-polio syndrome.

   a. _____

   b. _____

   c. _____

   d. _____

   e. _____

   f. _____

   g. _____

   h. _____

5. List at least eight things the nursing assistant should monitor or care for in the post-polio patient who has had surgery.

   a. _____

   b. _____

   c. _____

   d. _____

   e. _____

   f. _____

   g. _____

   h. _____

6. List 10 things the nursing assistant must do in caring for a patient with ALS.

   a. _____

   b. _____

   c. _____

   d. _____

   e. _____

f. _____

g. _____

h. _____

i. _____

j. _____

7. List six observations that should be reported to the nurse when a patient has had a seizure.

a. _____

b. _____

c. _____

d. _____

e. _____

f. _____

8. List at least 10 conditions that cause autonomic dysreflexia.

a. _____

b. _____

c. _____

d. _____

e. _____

f. _____

g. _____

h. _____

i. _____

j. _____

9. List 10 signs and symptoms of autonomic dysreflexia.

a. _____

b. _____

c. _____

d. _____

e. _____

f. _____

g. _____

h. _____

i. _____

j. _____

10. What are two important goals of nursing care of a patient during a seizure?

    a. _____

    b. _____

11. What are three ways to prevent contractures in the patient who has a spinal cord injury?

    a. _____

    b. _____

    c. _____

12. What two techniques can be learned to help communicate with someone who is deaf?

    a. _____

    b. _____

13. Complete the chart.

Type of Seizure	Description
a. absence	_____
b. generalized tonic-clonic	_____
c. status epilepticus	_____

True/False

Mark the following true or false by circling T or F.

1. T   F   Patients who are paralyzed are prone to pressure ulcers.

2. T   F   The ear mold of a hearing aid is removed by lifting the mold upward and outward.

3. T   F   During a seizure, an airway is best maintained by keeping the head straight.

4. T   F   Parkinson's disease is characterized by muscular rigidity and akinesia.

5. T   F   Intention tremors become worse as the individual tries to touch or pick up an object.

6. T   F   Multiple sclerosis is a progressive disease associated with inadequate levels of neurotransmitters in the cerebellum and brainstem.

7. T   F   Seizure syndrome is sometimes known as epilepsy.

8. T   F   Patients with spinal cord injuries need long-term nursing care.

9. T   F   Meningitis is an inflammation of the inner ear that may result in deafness.

Matching

Match the words on the right with the statements on the left.

1. _____ 3 percent of strokes; blood fills the space surrounding the brain rather than inside of it.

2. _____ Usually in the basal ganglia and thalamus; common in persons with diabetes and/or hypertension.

3. _____ Clot forms in the brain; usually in a cerebral artery.

4. _____ Sudden rupture of an artery; blood spills out, compressing brain structures.

5. _____ Temporary period of diminished blood flow to the brain; precedes 15 percent of all strokes.

6. _____ Most common type of stroke; about 87 percent of all strokes.

7. _____ Clot develops elsewhere in the body, then travels to brain and lodges in small artery.

a. Cerebral hemorrhage

b. Embolic stroke

c. Ischemic stroke

d. Lacunar infarct

e. Subarachnoid hemorrhage

f. Thrombotic stroke

g. Transient ischemic attack

Clinical Situations

Briefly describe how a nursing assistant should react to the following situations.

1. The patient is on the floor convulsing.

   _____

   _____

   _____

2. You notice a change in the level of consciousness of your patient with a head injury.

   _____

   _____

   _____

3. Your patient in the private room has post-polio syndrome. The bed is on the opposite wall of the room from her bed at home. She is having trouble getting into and out of bed.

   _____

   _____

   _____

4. Mr. Herrera, an ALS patient, had difficulty swallowing his regular diet when you fed him. He kept coughing and choking.

   _____

   _____

   _____

RELATING TO THE NURSING PROCESS

Write the step of the nursing process that is related to the nursing assistant action.

Nursing Assistant Action	Nursing Process Step
1. The nursing assistant notes uncontrolled body movements in the patient with a head injury and calls this to the nurse's attention.	_____
2. The nursing assistant helps the nurse turn and position the patient who has had a stroke.	_____
3. The nursing assistant carries out ROM exercises for the patient who is paralyzed.	_____
4. The nursing assistant finds a patient who is convulsing. She calls for help but does not leave the patient alone.	_____
5. The nursing assistant uses a picture board to assist in communication with a patient who has aphasia.	_____
6. The nursing assistant pays particular attention when the patient with Parkinson's disease ambulates, knowing that he is more apt to fall.	_____
7. The nursing assistant and all staff members try to maintain a calm environment for the patients with Parkinson's disease.	_____

DEVELOPING GREATER INSIGHT

1. Put cotton balls in your ears and try to communicate with your classmates. Discuss your feelings and frustrations.

2. Try communicating your feelings and needs to a classmate without words and without the use of one hand and arm. Describe your feelings.

Gastrointestinal System

OBJECTIVES

After completing this unit, you will be able to:

- Spell and define terms.
- Review the location and functions of the organs of the gastrointestinal system.
- List specific diagnostic tests associated with disorders of the gastrointestinal system.
- Describe some common disorders of the gastrointestinal system.
- Describe nursing assistant actions related to the care of patients with disorders of the gastrointestinal system.
- Identify different types of enemas and state their purpose.
- List the guidelines for caring for an ostomy.
- Demonstrate the following procedures:

  Procedure 110   Collecting a Stool Specimen

  Procedure 111   Testing for Occult Blood Using Hemoccult and Developer

  Procedure 112   Inserting a Rectal Suppository

  Procedure 113   Giving a Soap-Solution Enema

  Procedure 114   Giving a Commercially Prepared Enema

  Procedure 115   Inserting a Rectal Tube and Flatus Bag

  Procedure 116   Giving Routine Stoma Care (Colostomy)

  Procedure 117   Routine Care of an Ileostomy (with Patient in Bed)

UNIT SUMMARY

The organs in the digestive system are very complex. Because of their complexity, disease of these organs is fairly common. Common conditions include:

- Hernias

- Inflammation such as cholecystitis
- Cancer
- Ulcerations

Procedures performed on this system include:

- Enemas. Enemas are also performed before surgery on other parts of the body.

- Insertion of rectal tubes to relieve flatus.

- Insertion of rectal suppositories.

Great care must be exercised when performing the procedures. Remember that the patient's comfort and privacy should be protected at all times.

NURSING ASSISTANT ALERT

Action

Provide adequate coverage and privacy.

Maintain a matter-of-fact attitude.

Prepare patients for tests according to orders.

Benefit

Diminishes patient anxiety and embarrassment.

Protects patient's self-esteem.

Ensures more successful testing.

ACTIVITIES

Vocabulary Exercise

In the figure, put a circle around the word defined.

c	f	c	o	l	o	s	t	o	m	y	e	v	j	u
f	h	l	v	t	i	c	b	v	x	h	m	e	r	e
a	j	o	a	c	g	u	g	y	t	q	f	g	u	g
z	f	p	l	t	z	z	d	y	b	y	e	e	g	v
d	y	x	z	e	u	x	p	s	m	n	a	f	p	i
j	t	h	h	i	c	s	d	o	c	f	h	o	i	j
f	u	i	w	v	o	y	t	y	b	y	j	n	e	t
a	j	i	e	p	m	c	s	g	z	u	y	b	s	a
i	t	u	r	w	e	a	k	t	a	x	p	j	h	n
n	l	q	e	r	s	p	t	k	e	s	r	m	u	o
r	w	w	t	u	e	z	b	x	a	c	t	h	h	l
e	g	s	x	v	t	b	z	l	t	m	t	r	k	o
h	a	y	p	f	a	p	t	k	k	e	u	o	i	c
g	i	m	p	a	c	t	i	o	n	f	q	r	m	c
l	r	g	c	n	o	i	t	a	c	e	f	e	d	y

1. Removal of a gall bladder

2. Removal of the stomach

3. Artificial opening made in the large bowel for fecal elimination

4. Eliminating feces through the anus

5. Another name for the large bowel

6. Protrusion of the intestines through a weakened area in the abdominal wall

7. Collection of hardened feces in the rectum

8. Intestinal gas

9. A strong feeling of the need to eliminate

10. Pertaining to the stomach

Definitions

Define the following terms or abbreviations.

1. HCl

   _____

2. cholelithiasis

   _____

3. peristalsis

   _____

4. herniorrhaphy

   _____

5. impaction

   _____

6. bolus

   _____

7. umami

   _____

8. inguinal

   _____

9. papillae

   _____

10. TWE

   _____

Anatomy Review

Using colored pencils or crayons, color the organs of the digestive system as indicated.

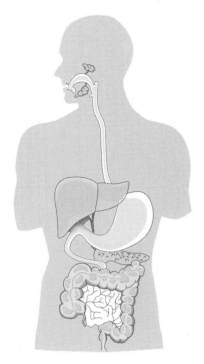

1. esophagus—blue

2. stomach—yellow

3. small intestine—green

4. liver—red

5. gallbladder—black

6. colon—blue

7. appendix—brown

8. pancreas—blue

Completion

Complete the following statements in the spaces provided.

1. An _____ of the gastrointestinal tract is often the first major sign
   of a tumor.

2. If a patient has a nasogastric tube in place, you must be careful when moving the patient to prevent
   _____.

3. Following a bowel resection, it may be necessary to create an artificial opening called a
   _____.

4. The patient with ulcerative colitis becomes dehydrated because of frequent _____.

5. The patient with ulcerative colitis should be eating a high-protein, high-calorie, _____
   diet.

6. The patient with a duodenal ulcer is given medication to neutralize the _____ of the stomach, which causes additional trauma to the _____ area.

7. If a patient has an NPO order, special _____ should be given.

8. The patient with cholecystitis or cholelithiasis is usually placed on a low- _____ diet.

9. Following a cholecystectomy, _____ are often placed in the operative area.

10. In addition to routine postoperative care, the cholecystectomy patient should be placed in the _____ position.

11. Your patient is scheduled for a GB series, so you should check for orders regarding _____ or a special _____.

12. The solution used for a soap-solution enema is _____.

13. The best patient position for administration of an enema is the _____.

14. When possible, an enema should be given _____ giving the bath.

15. A _____ is required before giving an enema.

16. An oil-retention enema is retained and followed with a _____ enema.

17. The lubricated enema tube should be inserted _____ into the anus.

18. The enema solution container should be raised _____ above the level of the _____ while allowing the fluid to flow into the patient.

19. Reusable enema equipment should be rinsed in _____ water before washing.

20. The rectal tube is used to relieve abdominal _____.

21. Commercially prepared chemical enema solutions drain fluid from the body to stimulate _____.

22. The chemical enema solution should be retained as _____.

23. Rectal tubes should be used no more than _____ in 24 hours.

24. Standard precautions require the use of _____ to protect the _____ from contamination during procedures involving the anus or rectum.

25. Antibiotics are given to control _____ that is involved in the development of gastric ulcers.

Short Answer

Briefly answer the following questions.

1. What are three important observations regarding your patient who has had a cholecystectomy that should immediately be reported to the nurse?

   a. _____

   b. _____

   c. _____

2. List 10 factors that affect bowel function and increase the risk of constipation.

   a. _____

   b. _____

   c. _____

d. _____

e. _____

f. _____

g. _____

h. _____

i. _____

j. _____

3. List at least 10 signs and symptoms of fecal impaction.

a. _____

b. _____

c. _____

d. _____

e. _____

f. _____

g. _____

h. _____

i. _____

j. _____

4. What are five reasons that enemas are commonly given?

a. _____

b. _____

c. _____

d. _____

e. _____

5. What information should be included when documenting an enema?

a. _____

b. _____

c. _____

d. _____

Clinical Situations

Briefly describe how a nursing assistant should react to the following situations.

1. You have an order to give a soap-solution enema and the patient has just finished breakfast.

_____

_____

2. The patient complains of cramping while you are giving an enema.

_____

_____

3. Your patient has returned from surgery following a cholecystectomy. Drains are in place.

_____

_____

4. Your patient expresses concern about retaining a rectal suppository.

_____

_____

RELATING TO THE NURSING PROCESS

Write the step of the nursing process that is related to the nursing assistant action.

Nursing Assistant Action	Nursing Process Step
1. The nursing assistant carefully explains the procedure before administering an enema to the patient.	_____
2. The nursing assistant inserts a lubricating suppository beyond the rectal sphincter.	_____
3. The nursing assistant instructs the patient that an oil-retention enema must be retained for at least 20 minutes after introduction.	_____
4. The nursing assistant lubricates the tip of the enema tube well before insertion.	_____
5. The nursing assistant reports and records the results of the soap-solution enema.	_____

DEVELOPING GREATER INSIGHT

1. Tumors of the colon can often grow large before being detected. Give some reasons why you think this might be.

_____

_____

2. Discuss reasons why enemas are given before a meal rather than after.

_____

_____

Urinary System

OBJECTIVES

After completing this unit, you will be able to:

- Spell and define terms.
- Review the location and function of the urinary system.
- List five diagnostic tests associated with conditions of the urinary system.
- Describe some common diseases of the urinary system.
- Describe nursing assistant actions related to the care of patients with urinary system diseases and conditions.
- State the purpose of renal dialysis and give an overview of two types of dialysis.
- Describe the care of a person with an indwelling catheter.
- State the reasons for removing an indwelling catheter as soon as possible.
- Demonstrate the following procedures:

  Procedure 118 Collecting a Routine Urine Specimen

  Procedure 119 Collecting a Clean-Catch Urine Specimen

  Procedure 120 Collecting a 24-Hour Urine Specimen

  Procedure 121 Collecting a Urine Specimen Through a Drainage Port

  Procedure 122 Routine Drainage Check

  Procedure 123 Giving Indwelling Catheter Care

  Procedure 124 Emptying a Urinary Drainage Unit

  Procedure 125 Disconnecting the Catheter

  Procedure 126 Applying a Condom for Urinary Drainage

  Procedure 127 Connecting a Catheter to a Leg Bag

  Procedure 128 Emptying a Leg Bag

  Procedure 129 Removing an Indwelling Catheter

4. The nursing assistant wears gloves when handling the patient's urinary drainage equipment. _____

5. The nursing assistant strains all urine as ordered when the patient has renal calculi. _____

6. If the patient is not circumcised, the nursing assistant makes sure to reposition the foreskin after giving indwelling catheter care. _____

7. The nursing assistant maintains a positive attitude when changing the soiled linen of a patient who is incontinent. _____

8. The nursing assistant uses standard precautions to collect and measure a urine specimen. _____

9. All the nursing assistants add urine to a 24-hour collection from a single patient even though the patient is the primary responsibility of one nursing assistant. _____

DEVELOPING GREATER INSIGHT

1. Discuss with classmates why continence is so important to self-esteem.

2. Discuss with classmates why gloves are to be worn when handling bedpans or urine samples.

Reproductive System

OBJECTIVES

After completing this unit, you will be able to:

- Spell and define terms.
- Review the location and functions of the organs of the male and female reproductive systems.
- Describe some common disorders and conditions of the male reproductive system.
- Describe some common disorders and conditions of the female reproductive system.
- List six diagnostic tests associated with conditions of the male and female reproductive systems.
- Describe nursing assistant actions related to the care of patients with conditions and diseases of the reproductive system.
- State the nursing precautions required for patients who have sexually transmitted diseases.
- Demonstrate the following procedures:

  Procedure 130   Giving a Nonsterile Vaginal Douche

UNIT SUMMARY

- A knowledge of the normal male and female reproductive structures is important for the nursing assistant who wishes to understand the related nursing care.

- Disposable equipment available in many hospitals makes nursing care more convenient and safer for the patient.

- The nursing assistant must be understanding and patient when providing care for patients

who have reproductive problems, because any surgery on the reproductive organs may have a strong psychological effect on the patient.

- The nursing assistant must practice proper infection control when caring for patients who have sexually transmitted diseases.

NURSING ASSISTANT ALERT

Action	Benefit
Be alert to and report indications of infections or abnormalities of the reproductive tract.	Therapy that is started early can avert more extensive body damage.
Practice breast or testicular self-examination regularly.	Protects your own health.
Remember that there is a strong relationship between the reproductive system and sexual identity.	Contributes to accepting the individual as a sexual being.
Recognize that any threat to the reproductive organs has a strong psychological impact on an individual.	Allows staff to be supportive.

ACTIVITIES

Vocabulary Exercise

Complete the puzzle by filling in the missing letters of words found in this unit. Use the definitions to help you discover these words.

1. _ _ _ _ M _ _ _ _ _ _
2. _ _ _ _ _ _ E _ _ _
3. _ _ N _ _ _ _ _ _
4. _ _ S _ _ _ _ _ _ _
5. _ _ _ T _ _
6. _ _ _ R _ _
7. _ _ _ _ U _ _
8. _ A _ _ _ _
9. _ _ _ _ T _ _
10. _ _ _ _ _ _ I _ _
11. _ _ _ O _ _ _ _ _
12. _ _ N _ _ _ _

1. lining of the uterus
2. protrusion of rectum into vagina
3. external reproductive organs
4. excision of a breast
5. male sex glands
6. womb
7. term for fallopian tube
8. female organ of copulation
9. pouch that covers the testes
10. infertility
11. a sexually transmitted disease
12. inflammation of the vagina

Anatomy Review

Male Tract. **Using colored pencils or crayons, color the organs of the male reproductive tract as indicated. In red, trace the pathway of sperm; follow from origin to leaving the body.**

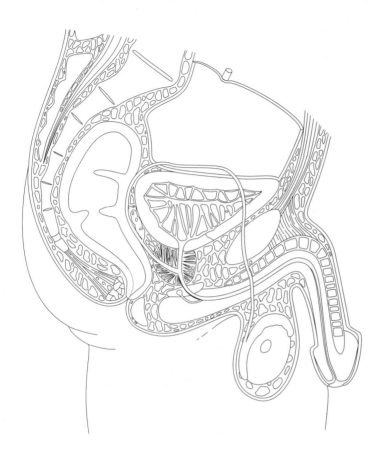

1. urinary bladder—yellow

2. penis—blue

3. testis—brown

4. prostate gland—green

Female Tract. **Using colored pencils or crayons, color the organs of the female tract as indicated. In red, trace the pathway of an egg from point of origin to uterus.**

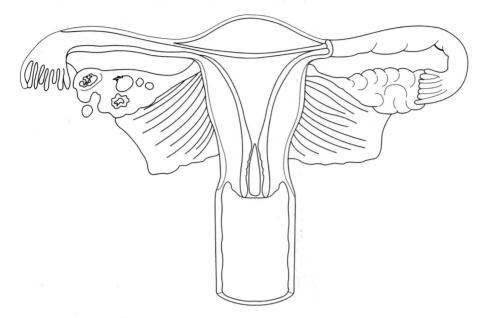

1. uterine walls—yellow

2. right ovary—blue

3. right oviduct—green

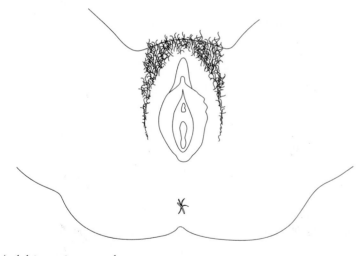

4. labia majora—red

5. clitoris—yellow

6. urinary meatus—green

7. labia minora—blue

Completion

Complete the statements in the spaces provided.

1. A common enlargement of the prostate gland is called benign _____.

2. The tube-like organ passing through the center of the prostate gland is the _____.

3. A major problem for men suffering from the condition named in question 1 is urinary _____.

4. Men undergoing prostatectomy are apt to be _____ upset by the thought of the procedure.

5. The patient who is returning from prostate surgery will have a _____ in place.

6. Testicular self-examination should be performed at least once each _____.

7. The best time to perform testicular self-examination is during a _____.

8. A colporrhaphy is performed to tighten the _____ walls.

9. An uncomfortable and distressing problem associated with a cystocele is urinary _____.

10. Vulvovaginitis that is often caused by *Candida albicans* is a/an _____ infection.

11. A simple test used to detect possible cancer of the cervix is the _____.

12. A _____ is a surgical procedure employed to help diagnose conditions of the uterus.

13. Removal of the fallopian tubes is known as a bilateral _____.

14. Following a mastectomy, bed linen should be checked, because blood may drain to the _____ of the dressing.

15. Vaginitis caused by *Trichomonas vaginalis* is associated with a foul-smelling discharge called _____.

16. In early stages, females infected with *Neisseria gonorrhea* are frequently _____ that they have been infected.

17. The organism that causes syphilis is known to pass from mother to child through the _____.

18. *Chlamydia* infections can cause serious _____.

19. Cancer of the testes may require removal by a surgical procedure called an _____.

20. Prostate cancer may be treated with _____, a procedure in which radioactive pellets are implanted.

21. Although viruses cannot be eliminated, medications are available to stop the _____ of the virus in patients with herpes.

22. HIV disease destroys the _____.

23. There is no _____ for HIV/AIDS, but drugs can slow the damage to the body.

24. A _____ occurs when the uterus slips downward into the vaginal canal.

25. A 2007 study found that _____, a little-known and difficult-to-detect STD, was more prevalent than gonorrhea in U.S. adolescents.

Short Answer

Briefly answer the following questions.

1. What three functions do the male and female reproductive tracts have in common?

    a. _____

    b. _____

    c. _____

2. What special care should you give postoperatively when caring for the patient who has had a prostatectomy?

   a. _____

   b. _____

   c. _____

   d. _____

   e. _____

   f. _____

   g. _____

   h. _____

   i. _____

   j. _____

3. Why is an attempt made to leave at least part of an ovary when a hysterectomy is needed in a younger woman?

_____

_____

4. When and how should a woman check her breasts?

   a. _____

   b. _____

5. How often should the procedure for testicular self-examination be performed?

   a. _____

6. What are two problems associated with rectoceles?

   a. _____

   b. _____

7. Why is it important to maintain good circulation in the patient who has just experienced a panhysterectomy?

_____

_____

8. What are six signs or symptoms of a breast tumor?

   a. _____

   b. _____

   c. _____

   d. _____

   e. _____

   f. _____

Clinical Situations

Briefly describe how a nursing assistant should react to the following situations.

1. A patient expresses concern about being able to perform sexually after brachytherapy for prostate cancer.

   _____

   _____

2. A patient is to have a lumpectomy and wants to know if the entire breast will be removed.

   _____

   _____

3. Your patient is scheduled for a suprapubic prostatectomy. He expresses to you his concerns about the possibility of being impotent following surgery.

   _____

   _____

RELATING TO THE NURSING PROCESS

Write the step of the nursing process that is related to the nursing assistant action.

Nursing Assistant Action	Nursing Process Step
1. The nursing assistant reports to the nurse that the patient is complaining of itching and has a watery vaginal discharge.	_____
2. The nursing assistant checks the bed at the patient's back for bleeding after the patient has had a mastectomy.	_____
3. The nursing assistant informs the nurse of the grief and frustrations the postoperative mastectomy patient is expressing.	_____
4. The nursing assistant inserts the douche nozzle slowly, while the fluid is flowing, in an upward and backward motion.	_____
5. The nursing assistant carefully notes and reports color and amount of drainage from all areas for the patient who has had a prostatectomy.	_____

DEVELOPING GREATER INSIGHT

1. Think about how you would feel if you found a lump in your breast or testes. What if it turned out to be malignant?

2. Discuss reasons why people tend to be particularly sensitive when there is disease or injury involving the reproductive organs.

3. Think about why it is important to use standard precautions when caring for patients who have sexually transmitted diseases.

Expanded Role of the Nursing Assistant

U N I T **47**

Caring for the Patient with Cancer

OBJECTIVES

After completing this unit, you will be able to:

- Spell and define terms.
- List methods of reducing the risk of cancer.
- Explain the importance of good nutrition in cancer prevention and treatment.
- List seven signs and symptoms of cancer.
- Describe three types of cancer treatment.
- Describe nursing assistant responsibilities when caring for patients with cancer.

UNIT SUMMARY

- Cancer cells grow abnormally, invade surrounding tissues, and use oxygen and nutrients targeted for normal cells.

- Some risk factors for cancer are genetic, but others are environmental. The American Cancer Society recommends some lifestyle changes and prevention measures.

- There is a direct relationship between intake of certain foods and the development of certain types of cancers.

- Regular cancer screening is key to survival, because the outcome is better if the disease is detected early.

- Many treatment options are used for cancer, including mainstream medicine, immunotherapy, drugs, radiation, surgery, and alternative and complementary therapies. Some treatments have very uncomfortable side effects.

- Pain is the most common symptom of patients with cancer.

- The nursing assistant should be prepared to support patients' emotional needs, and to provide physical care and comfort measures.

NURSING ASSISTANT ALERT

Action	Benefit
Ensure privacy, reduce noise, eliminate unpleasant odors, and adjust the temperature, lighting, and ventilation.	Reduces factors that cause discomfort over which the patient has no control.
	Makes the patient more comfortable.
Handle the patient gently, assist the patient to assume a comfortable position, use pillows and props for repositioning, give backrubs, and provide emotional support.	Helps the patient to relax and rest better.
	Enhances comfort.
Apply the principles of standard precautions and other infection control measures.	Reduces the risk of nosocomial infection.

ACTIVITIES

Vocabulary Exercise

Complete the puzzle.

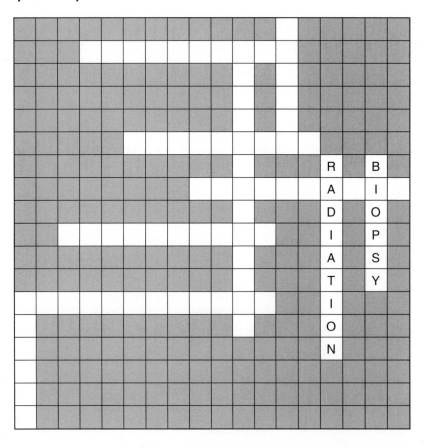

6 letters	**9 letters**	**10 letters**	**12 letters**	**13 letters**
BENIGN	MALIGNANT	CARCINOGEN	CHEMOTHERAPY	IMMUNOTHERAPY
BIOPSY	RADIATION	METASTASIS		
CANCER		PALLIATIVE		

Completion

Complete the following statements in the spaces provided.

1. Cancer is a disease in which the normal mechanisms of _____ are disturbed.

2. Cancer cells use the _____ and _____ targeted for normal cells.

3. Cancers that stay in one location and do not spread are _____.

4. Some types of cancer cells _____, or spread to other parts of the body through the blood and lymphatic systems.

5. Cancers that spread to other parts of the body are _____.

6. A _____ such as tobacco is a cancer-causing substance.

7. People with _____ warning signs of cancer should see a doctor right away.

8. Women should perform breast self-examination _____.

9. Men should perform _____ self-examination _____.

10. A _____ is a minor surgery that is sometimes done to remove tissue to diagnose cancer.

11. _____ involves the use of medications or drugs to destroy the cancer.

12. The nursing assistant should never _____, _____, or _____ in an area where chemotherapy is being prepared.

13. Waste products from some patients who are receiving chemotherapy require special _____.

14. _____ involves the use of high-energy, ionizing beams aimed at the site of the cancer.

15. _____ is a cancer treatment that alters the patient's immune response to eliminate the cancer.

16. Cancer patients' pain should be treated before it becomes _____.

Short Answer

Briefly complete the following.

1. List eight risk factors for cancer.

    a. _____

    b. _____

    c. _____

    d. _____

    e. _____

    f. _____

    g. _____

    h. _____

2. List four dietary guidelines that will help prevent cancer.

    a. _____

    b. _____

    c. _____

    d. _____

3. List seven lifestyle changes that will help prevent cancer.

    a. _____

    b. _____

    c. _____

    d. _____

    e. _____

    f. _____

    g. _____

4. Complete the following chart listing signs and symptoms of cancer.

    C = _____

    A = _____

    U = _____

    T = _____

    I = _____

    O = _____

    N = _____

5. List eight side effects of the drugs used to treat cancer.

    a. _____

    b. _____

    c. _____

    d. _____

    e. _____

    f. _____

    g. _____

    h. _____

6. List at least seven observations that should be reported to the nurse about patients who are receiving chemotherapy.

    a. _____

    b. _____

    c. _____

    d. _____

    e. _____

f. _____

g. _____

7. List eight side effects of radiation therapy that should be reported promptly to the nurse.

a. _____

b. _____

c. _____

d. _____

e. _____

f. _____

g. _____

h. _____

8. List five measures to take to protect yourself from exposure to radiation.

a. _____

b. _____

c. _____

d. _____

e. _____

9. List seven observations of the patient who is receiving immunotherapy to report to the nurse.

a. _____

b. _____

c. _____

d. _____

e. _____

f. _____

g. _____

10. List eight ways in which the nursing assistant can help meet patients' emotional needs.

a. _____

b. _____

c. _____

d. _____

e. _____

f. _____

g. _____

h. _____

True/False

Mark the following true or false by circling T or F.

1. T   F   Breast cancer, ovarian cancer, and pancreatic cancer seem to have a hereditary component.

2. T   F   Most cancers occur in individuals over the age of 45.

3. T   F   Obesity is associated with cancer of the brain and lungs.

4. T   F   Salt from all food sources should not exceed 3 teaspoons a day.

5. T   F   Surgery is sometimes done as a means of cancer prevention.

6. T   F   Although a cure may not be possible, chemotherapy is sometimes done to control and slow the growth of cancer to prolong the patient's life.

7. T   F   Wash your hands well if you contact a chemotherapy drug.

8. T   F   Side effects of some cancer treatments are life-threatening.

9. T   F   Good nutrition and hydration are not particularly important in cancer patients.

10. T   F   Hair loss is very upsetting to most people.

11. T   F   Shave the area surrounding the patient's radiation treatment field each day.

12. T   F   Vital signs should be closely monitored when immunotherapy is used.

13. T   F   Cancer treatment may be painful for the patient.

14. T   F   Cancer patients have a high incidence of addiction to narcotic pain-relieving drugs.

15. T   F   The nursing assistant should always try to instill hope in the patient.

16. T   F   Providing compassionate care, listening, and giving sincere, solid emotional support will help patients and family members cope with cancer.

17. T   F   Many cancer patients fear dying.

18. T   F   The WHO analgesic ladder is often used in the management of pain in cancer patients.

19. T   F   Itching is a side effect of immunotherapy.

20. T   F   Always take a rectal temperature for patients who are receiving chemotherapy.

21. T   F   Patients with cancer may go through the grieving process.

22. T   F   Monitor the chemotherapy patient for bleeding, bruising, and abnormal skin lesions.

23. T   F   Following radiation treatments, scrub the markings off the patient's body.

24. T   F   Palliative care is an aggressive cancer treatment.

25. T   F   All cancer patients have "do not resuscitate" orders.

RELATING TO THE NURSING PROCESS

Write the step of the nursing process that is related to the nursing assistant action.

Nursing Assistant Action	Nursing Process Step
1. The nursing assistant reports to the nurse that Mrs. Lichtenstein, the chemotherapy patient in 222, is vomiting and refused her supper tray.	_____
2. The nursing assistant reports in care conference that Lashanda Mauro, the cancer patient in 233-A, uses aromatherapy to help relieve her nausea.	_____
3. The nursing assistant informs the nurse that Mr. Ferraro's temperature is 102.6°F.	_____
4. The nursing assistant reports that the injection relieved the patient's pain.	_____
5. The nursing assistant followed the nurse's instructions to sit with the patient and listen to her until she calmed down.	_____

DEVELOPING GREATER INSIGHT

1. Ask a representative of the American Cancer Society or a cancer survivor to speak to the class.

2. Discuss with a group how you would feel if you were given a terminal cancer diagnosis today.

Rehabilitation and Restorative Services

OBJECTIVES

After completing this unit, you will be able to:

- Spell and define terms.
- Compare and contrast rehabilitation and restorative nursing care.
- Describe the role of the nursing assistant in rehabilitation and restorative care.
- Describe the principles of rehabilitation.
- List the elements of successful rehabilitation/restorative care.
- List six complications resulting from inactivity.
- Identify four perceptual deficits.
- Describe four approaches used for restorative programs.
- List guidelines for providing restorative care.
- Describe monitoring of the resident's response to care.

UNIT SUMMARY

Rehabilitation and restorative care are designed to help patients reach an optimal level of personal ability. The most successful programs:

- Begin as soon as possible.
- Stress ability and not disability.
- Treat the whole person.

Care is planned by an interdisciplinary health care team, of which the nursing assistant is an important member.

Nursing assistants participate in the restorative program by:

- Knowing and following the stated nursing health care plan
- Supporting the patient's efforts toward independence
- Assisting the nurses with procedures designed to meet specific patient needs
- Maintaining the patient's nutrition

Nursing assistants can make a valuable contribution to the success of the patient's program by demonstrating a consistent, positive, and patient attitude.

RELATING TO THE NURSING PROCESS

Write the step of the nursing process that is related to the nursing assistant action.

Nursing Assistant Action	Nursing Process Step
1. The nursing assistant begins passive exercises and positioning for Mrs. Burton, who is stable after a right-sided stroke.	_____
2. The nursing assistant encourages Mr. Jackson, who has poor strength in his dominant right hand, as he tries to feed himself with his left hand.	_____
3. The nursing assistant participates in team care conferences.	_____
4. The nursing assistant reports that Mrs. Parson is able to move her hands but is unable to select and hold items.	_____

DEVELOPING GREATER INSIGHT

1. With a classmate acting as a nursing assistant, practice trying to use your nondominant hand to eat, secure your shoes, and put on your clothes. Discuss how it makes you feel.

2. When first waking in the morning, lie in bed and think how frustrating it would be not to be able to carry out your morning hygiene routine.

3. Borrow a wheelchair and try to navigate around your community, home, and school campus. Discuss the problems you encounter when you cannot use your legs to walk.

Obstetrical Patients and Neonates

OBJECTIVES

After completing this unit, you will be able to:

- Spell and define terms.
- Define *doula* and identify the role and responsibilities of the doula as a member of the childbirth team.
- Assist in care of the normal postpartum patient.
- Properly change a perineal pad.
- Recognize reportable observations of patients in the postpartum period.
- Assist in care of the normal newborn.
- Demonstrate three methods of safely holding a baby.
- Describe nursing assistant actions and observations related to the care of the newborn infant.
- List measures to prevent inadvertent switching, misidentification, and abduction of infants.
- Assist in carrying out the discharge procedures for mother and infant.
- Demonstrate the following procedures:

  Procedure 131   Changing a Diaper

  Procedure 132   Weighing the Infant

  Procedure 133   Measuring the Infant

  Procedure 134   Bathing an Infant

  Procedure 135   Bottle-Feeding an Infant

  Procedure 136   Assisting with Breast Feeding

  Procedure 137   Burping an Infant

UNIT SUMMARY

The care of the obstetrical patient is a very specialized area of medicine. It includes:

- Supervision of the mother's health throughout the prenatal, labor and delivery, and postpartum periods to discharge.

- Care of the neonate.

The nursing assistant may participate in this care under the close direction of the professional staff if facility policy permits.

A thorough understanding of your responsibilities and close attention to the details of care help ensure a successful and safe pregnancy and delivery.

All the procedures presented in this unit require advanced training and supervision before you attempt to perform them. In addition, you may do so only with proper authorization and under proper supervision.

NURSING ASSISTANT ALERT

Action	Benefit
Follow orders carefully during the prenatal, delivery, and postpartum periods.	Helps ensure a successful and safe pregnancy and delivery.
Keep one hand near the baby when weighing it.	Prevents injury to the infant.
Handle and carry babies securely in an approved manner.	Protects the baby from injury.
Be open with and supportive of parents who are faced with difficult or unsuccessful pregnancies and deliveries.	Provides essential emotional support when parents need it the most.

ACTIVITIES

Vocabulary Exercise

Each line has four different spellings of a word. Circle the correctly spelled word.

1. lokia   lochia   lokeya   lochea

2. neonat   nionat   nionate   neonate

3. fetis   feetes   fetus   feitas

4. doola   duela   doula   doolle

5. umbalical   umbilicale   umbilical   umbelical

6. isolette   eyesolet   isoullette   aecollet

7. arreala   airiola   aerealla   areola

8. preenatul   prenatal   preanatul   prenattel

Definitions

Define the following terms.

1. amniotic sac _____

2. umbilical cord _____

3. postpartum _____

4. lactation _____

5. neonate _____

6. placenta _____

Completion

Complete the following statements in the spaces provided.

1. A clinic that provides care during and following pregnancy is called a/an _____ clinic.

2. After the baby is born, the placenta, amniotic sac, and remaining cord are expelled as the _____.

3. When taking the vital signs in the first few hours after a woman gives birth, position the mother _____.

4. Position the mother _____ if spinal anesthesia was used.

5. Immediately after birth, monitor the mother's vital signs every _____ for _____.

6. Lift the peri pad away from the body from _____ to _____.

7. The lochia is initially _____ in color.

8. _____ occurs when the uterus begins to return to normal size.

9. Instruct the mother to _____ before flushing the toilet.

10. Foul-smelling lochia is a sign of _____.

11. Teach the mother to use anesthetic spray _____ cleansing the perineum.

12. The part of the mother's milk that carries important, protective antibodies to the infant is called _____.

13. While weighing a baby, never turn your _____ to the scale, and keep one _____ over the baby at all times.

14. If it is necessary to carry the infant in your arms, always _____ through a doorway.

15. Be sure to wash hands _____ and _____ handling each child and after each _____ change.

16. A circumcision should be checked _____.

17. _____, also known as the flow of milk, does not begin until the _____.

18. The baby is dressed in _____ clothes for discharge.

19. A new mother should be encouraged to void within the first _____ hours postpartum.

20. Teach the mother to handle the peri pad only _____.

21. When removing a soiled perineal pad, the nursing assistant must always wear _____,
fold the soiled side of the pad _____, and wrap the pad in a _____.

22. Never dispose of soiled perineal pads in the _____.

23. Mothers who are breastfeeding should be instructed to wash their breasts using a
_____ motion from _____ to outward.

24. The Apgar score is an evaluation of the _____ which is made at
_____ minute and _____ minutes after birth.

25. An Apgar score of 9 indicates that the neonate is in _____ condition.

26. The baby must be kept warm until its _____ stabilizes.

27. In the nursery, the _____, weight, and vital signs are measured.

28. The infant can lose a great deal of body heat through the _____.

29. The _____ is responsible for supporting and comforting the mother and enhancing
communication between the mother and medical professionals.

Short Answer

Briefly answer the following questions.

1. What three techniques might be ordered to relieve the perineal discomfort of an episiotomy?

    a. _____

    b. _____

    c. _____

2. What is the primary value of colostrum to the baby?

    a. _____

    b. _____

3. What is the purpose of Apgar scoring?

    _____

4. List ways of caring for the breast of the nursing mother.

    a. _____

    b. _____

    c. _____

    d. _____

    e. _____

5. How should the baby be lifted from the crib?

    a. _____

    b. _____

Clinical Situations

Briefly explain how the nursing assistant should react to the following situations.

1. The new mother is very uncomfortable when she tries to sit. _____

   _____

   _____

2. The new mother has returned to your care in the postpartum area.

   a. _____

   b. _____

   c. _____

   d. _____

   e. _____

Identification

1. Write the names of the parts or structures indicated in the spaces provided.

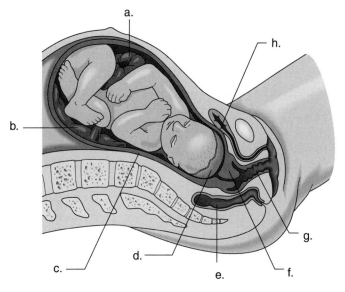

   a. _____

   b. _____

   c. _____

   d. _____

   e. _____

   f. _____

   g. _____

   h. _____

RELATING TO THE NURSING PROCESS

Write the step of the nursing process that is related to the nursing assistant action.

Nursing Assistant Action   **Nursing Process Step**

1. The nursing assistant helps other staff members
   transfer the mother who has just given birth from
   stretcher to bed.   _____

2. The nursing assistant checks the mother's vital signs
   as ordered following a cesarean section.   _____

3. The nursing assistant measures and records the first
   postpartum voiding.   _____

4. The nursing assistant instructs the mother to stand up
   before flushing the toilet.   _____

DEVELOPING GREATER INSIGHT

1. Identify what special help a new mother may require because she does not remain in the hospital very long
   for care.

2. Invite someone from a maternity department to speak to the class about how to prevent infant abduction.

Pediatric Patients

After completing this unit, you will be able to:

- Spell and define terms.
- Describe how to foster the growth and development of hospitalized pediatric patients.
- Describe how to maintain a safe environment for the pediatric patient.
- Discuss the problem of childhood obesity and identify special problems and complications that occur as a result of this condition.
- Discuss the role of parents and siblings of the hospitalized pediatric patient.
- Describe Munchausen by proxy syndrome (MBPS).
- List signs and symptoms of physical, emotional, and sexual abuse and neglect.
- Demonstrate the following procedures:

  Procedure 138   Admitting a Pediatric Patient

  Procedure 139   Weighing the Toddler to Adolescent

  Procedure 140   Changing Crib Linens

  Procedure 141   Changing Crib Linens (Infant in Crib)

  Procedure 142   Measuring Temperature

  Procedure 143   Determining Heart Rate (Pulse)

  Procedure 144   Counting Respiratory Rate

  Procedure 145   Measuring Blood Pressure

  Procedure 146   Collecting a Urine Specimen from an Infant

UNIT SUMMARY

This unit provides the nursing assistant with information on giving safe care to the hospitalized pediatric patient. Because children differ in age, size, and developmental level, five developmental levels are described:

- Infancy
- Toddlerhood
- Preschooler
- School-age
- Adolescence

For each age group, suggestions are offered to promote normal growth and development while maintaining a safe environment for the hospitalized pediatric patient.

Families are important to the pediatric patient. Because the family can also be affected by the child's hospitalization, suggestions are provided to promote and encourage a family-centered approach to care.

NURSING ASSISTANT ALERT

Action	Benefit
Maintain a safe environment.	Keeps the child safe from injury.
Provide opportunities for decision making.	Supports the child's need for growing independence.
Familiarize yourself with the usual changes that occur at different chronological ages.	Recognize that people reach developmental stages at different rates.
	Helps to ensure individualization of patient care.

ACTIVITIES

Vocabulary Exercise

1. In the figure, put a circle around the word defined.

r	p	e	d	i	a	t	r	i	c	p	i	d
f	e	r	e	g	r	e	s	s	c	n	e	z
a	o	t	l	s	v	b	z	w	f	v	j	c
n	j	a	s	e	x	s	c	a	e	c	q	e
t	e	y	d	o	c	v	n	l	y	t	s	g
a	t	y	p	o	f	t	o	i	d	i	g	a
s	a	s	r	o	l	p	o	t	b	j	n	~
i	i	r	s	n	m	e	b	l	x	t	i	l
e	v	x	c	e	e	i	s	q	z	r	l	o
s	e	p	n	s	z	a	p	c	e	c	b	o
l	d	t	x	j	r	o	o	f	e	x	i	h
u	a	d	h	y	x	o	h	r	k	n	s	c
l	u	k	y	m	o	n	o	t	u	a	t	s

a. magical thinking

b. to promote

c. brothers and sisters

d. to move backward

e. a child from birth to 1 year

f. to move away from center

g. children from 6 to 12 years

h. children from 13 to 18 years

i. pertaining to children

j. able to make choices independently

k. intellectual, social, and emotional tasks that must be accomplished at a certain age level

Completion

Complete the statements in the spaces provided.

1. What are two ways pediatric departments are usually organized?

   a. _____

   b. _____

2. Who provides the medical and social history when the patient is a child?

   _____

   _____

3. How will the infant change in the first year of life?

   a. _____

   b. _____

4. What is meant by the infant's "developmental milestones"?

   _____

   _____

5. What is the primary psychosocial development task for the infant?

   _____

   _____

6. How might you foster achievement of the infant's developmental task?

   _____

   _____

7. How should the care of an infant be organized?

   _____

   _____

8. If a toddler is unable to stand on an upright scale, how may he be weighed?

_____

_____

9. What factors would increase the infant's heart rate and respirations?

a. _____

b. _____

c. _____

10. List the sequence for taking vital signs on an infant when a rectal temperature is to be measured.

_____

_____

11. How might an infant's sucking needs be met when she cannot eat?

_____

_____

12. If the toddler is toilet trained, what information would be helpful for you to know?

_____

_____

13. What is a major fear of the preschooler?

_____

_____

14. Because preschoolers have a limited concept of time, how should you explain when something will occur?

_____

_____

15. How could you foster a school-age child's need for accomplishment?

_____

_____

16. How may an adolescent view the nursing assistant and other caregivers?

_____

_____

17. Who are the most important people to the adolescent?

_____

_____

18. When using a tympanic thermometer to take an infant or child's temperature, what should the nursing assistant do to ensure an accurate reading?

_____

_____

19. How would you obtain a urine specimen from a 6-month old infant who wears a diaper and has good skin integrity?

_____

_____

20. List five signs or symptoms of child abuse.

    a. _____

    b. _____

    c. _____

    d. _____

    e. _____

21. Describe Munchausen by proxy syndrome (MBPS).

    _____

    _____

22. How does the caregiver treat the Munchausen by proxy syndrome (MBPS) child?

    _____

    _____

23. Altered appearance upsets teenagers' feelings about their _____.

24. The abused child lives in an _____ world and feels constant _____.

True/False

Mark the following true or false by circling T or F.

1. T F   When a child is hospitalized, caregivers may assume the role of substitute mother.

2. T F   A 6-month-old infant is able to sit well and pull herself into a standing position.

3. T F   Infants do not normally respond to voices, faces, or touch of strangers.

4. T F   The radial pulse is used for counting the pulse in an infant.

5. T F   Blood pressure is not routinely taken in infants and small children.

6. T F   A sterile bottle, nipple, and formula are necessary when feeding an infant.

7. T F   It is not necessary to burp an infant until the infant has consumed the entire bottle.

8. T F   It is best to restrain toddlers by keeping them in bed to prevent injury.

9. T F   The caregiver always advocates for the child in cases of MBPS.

10. T F   The MSBP caregivers derive self-esteem and satisfaction by misleading health care providers whom they consider to be much more important and powerful than themselves.

11. T F   As a rule, the MSBP caregiver is unable to deceive health care professionals.

12. T F   The mother is responsible for causing MSBP in 47 percent of all cases.

13. T F   Toddlers are too immature to need autonomy.

14. T F   Toddlers usually do not handle separation from the mother well.

15. T F   Finger painting is a good activity for toddlers.

16. T F   Allow the 6-year-old to do as much of his own care as possible.

17. T F   It is not necessary to explain procedures to school-age children.

18. T F   School-age children do not need privacy during personal care procedures.

19. T F Games are a good activity for the school-age child.

20. T F Body image is not important to adolescents.

21. T F A safe environment is not a concern for adolescent patients.

22. T F Allow adolescents to have as much control over their routines as possible.

Clinical Situations

Briefly describe how a nursing assistant should react to the following situations.

1. The toddler who is weaned cries for a bottle. _____

_____

_____

2. The toddler is having a temper tantrum. _____

_____

_____

3. The teenager does not want to go to sleep after the television has been shut off.

_____

_____

_____

RELATING TO THE NURSING PROCESS

Write the step of the nursing process that is related to the nursing assistant action.

Nursing Assistant Action	Nursing Process Step
1. The nursing assistant measures and weighs the child during admission to the pediatric unit.	_____
2. The nursing assistant helps stabilize the preschooler's arm while offering comforting support during blood withdrawal.	_____
3. The nursing assistant finds ways to occupy a roommate when a school-age patient is visited by a tutor.	_____
4. The nursing assistant always keeps the crib sides up when the toddler is in the crib.	_____
5. The nursing assistant discusses with the nurse about activities for the recuperating toddler in her care.	_____

DEVELOPING GREATER INSIGHT

1. Describe as many different types of "family units" as you can.

2. Discuss reasons why teens join gangs. How will you feel about caring for a teen who was injured in a gang fight?

Response to Basic Emergencies

Response to Basic Emergencies

OBJECTIVES

After completing this unit, you will be able to:

- Spell and define terms.

- Recognize emergency situations that require urgent care.

- Evaluate situations and determine the sequence of appropriate actions to be taken.

- List and describe the 11 standardized types of codes.

- Describe how to maintain the patient's airway and breathing during respiratory failure and respiratory arrest.

- Recognize the need for CPR.

- List the benefits of early defibrillation.

- Identify the signs, symptoms, and treatment of common emergency situations such as:

  Cardiac arrest

  Choking

  Bleeding

  Shock

  Fainting

Heart attack

Brain attack (stroke)

Seizure

Vomiting and aspiration

Thermal injuries

Poisoning

Known or suspected head injury

- Demonstrate the following procedures:

    Procedure 147   Head-Tilt, Chin-Lift Maneuver

    Procedure 148   Jaw-Thrust Maneuver

    Procedure 149   Mask-to-Mouth Ventilation

    Procedure 150   Positioning the Patient in the Recovery Position

    Procedure 151   Assisting the Adult Who Has an Obstructed Airway and Becomes Unconscious

    Procedure 152   Obstructed Airway: Infant

    Procedure 153   Child with Foreign Body Airway Obstruction

UNIT SUMMARY

Emergency situations can occur without warning at any time. A person who has been specially trained in the techniques of first aid can be of great service.

- Remain calm.

- Know the correct standardized code words to use to get the correct type of response.

- Remain with the patient (unless otherwise instructed) until further help arrives, and perform any emergency procedures that you are qualified and permitted to do.

- Never overestimate your abilities.

- Use the special skills you have been taught wisely.

Special training will enable you to assess injuries and know the proper steps to follow in:

- Calling for help.

- Carrying out lifesaving skills.

- Controlling bleeding.

- Helping victims of accidents and injuries.

NURSING ASSISTANT ALERT

Action	Benefit
Never overestimate your abilities.	Prevents injuries due to improper actions.
Follow only approved actions.	Can be lifesaving. Avoids legal liability.

ACTIVITIES

Vocabulary Exercise

Complete the puzzle by filling in the missing letters of words found in this unit. Use the definitions to help you discover these words.

1.	_ _ _ U _ _	1. Injury
2.	_ _ R _ _ _	2. Stoppage of heartbeat
3.	_ _ _ _ _ _ _ G	3. Sudden loss of consciousness
4.	_ _ _ _ _ E _ _	4. An unintended occurrence
5.	_ _ _ _ _ _ N _ _	5. A situation that develops rapidly and unexpectedly
6.	_ _ _ _ T _ _ _ _ _ _	6. Emergency cardiac condition
7.	_ _ _ _ C _	7. Disturbance of oxygen supply to the tissues and return of blood to heart
8.	_ _ _ _ A _ _	8. To raise
9.	_ _ R	9. Cardiopulmonary resuscitation
10.	_ E _ _ _ _ _ _ _ _	10. Loss of large amount of blood

Completion

Complete the statements in the spaces provided.

1. Your actions should never place the victim in additional _____.

2. First aid techniques are taught as a specific course by the _____.

3. Certification in CPR is provided in courses by the _____ and the American Red Cross.

4. In an emergency situation, always defer to someone who has greater _____ or _____.

5. When you provide first aid, you must deal with the victim's _____ as well as the victim's physical injuries.

6. The first step when arriving at the scene of an accident is to _____ the situation.

7. If you are in a medical facility when an accident occurs, you should _____ for help and keep the patient _____.

8. The national number for emergency help is _____.

9. The most common cause of airway obstruction is _____, so pulling the _____ forward often opens the airway.

10. If oxygen is denied to the body, the most sensitive organ, the _____, may suffer permanent damage.

11. The compression-to-ventilation ratio for CPR is _____ compressions to _____ ventilations.

12. Care that must be given immediately to prevent loss of life is called _____.

13. When moving a victim, always move him as a single _____.

14. The Heimlich maneuver refers to the technique of performing _____ thrusts.

15. Finger sweeps should only be used if you can _____ a foreign body in the victim's throat or mouth.

16. A disturbance of the oxygen supply to the tissues and return of blood to the heart is defined as _____.

17. The victim who is in shock should be kept _____ down.

18. The loss of heart function is called _____.

19. Seizures do not always follow the same _____.

20. In a generalized tonic-clonic (grand mal) seizure, the patient must be protected against _____ himself.

21. Following a generalized tonic-clonic (grand mal) seizure, the patient may be _____ and _____ for a time and feel very tired.

22. A good way to move a victim of electric shock away from the source of electricity is to use something made of _____.

Short Answer

Briefly answer the following questions.

1. What four basic actions should be taken in all emergency situations?

    a. _____

    b. _____

    c. _____

    d. _____

2. What facts should be included when calling the emergency number?

    a. _____

    b. _____

    c. _____

    d. _____

    e. _____

3. What two types of care are included in first aid?

    a. _____

    b. _____

4. What is the purpose of having standardized code words? _____

_____

_____

_____

_____

5. What are three ways to summon help for an accident victim in a health facility?

   a. _____

   b. _____

   c. _____

6. How should you check for breathing activity?

   a. _____

   b. _____

7. What order of victim's responses should be checked when providing urgent care?

   a. _____

   b. _____

   c. _____

8. How would you describe the distress signals of choking?

   _____

   _____

9. What steps should you follow to prevent additional blood loss in a bleeding victim?

   a. _____

   b. _____

   c. _____

   d. _____

   e. _____

   f. _____

10. What are the early signs of shock?

    a. _____

    b. _____

    c. _____

    d. _____

    e. _____

11. What signs and symptoms might indicate that the victim is having a heart attack?

    a. _____

    b. _____

    c. _____

    d. _____

    e. _____

Clinical Situations

Briefly describe how a nursing assistant should react to the following situations.

1. You are the first person on the scene of an auto accident. One person has been thrown out of the car and is lying beside the car, which is on fire. Describe your first action.

   _____

   _____

   _____

2. You discover the husband of your home client on the floor of the basement near a frayed electrical wire. What is your first action?

   _____

   _____

   _____

3. You are in a dining area when an ambulatory patient grasps his throat and is unable to speak.

   _____

   _____

   _____

RELATING TO THE NURSING PROCESS

Write the step of the nursing process that is related to the nursing assistant action.

Nursing Assistant Action	Nursing Process Step
1. The nursing assistant, finding a patient on the floor, first checks for consciousness.	_____
2. The nursing assistant finds an unconscious patient and immediately signals for help.	_____
3. The patient stumbles, injuring her knee, which begins to bleed. The nursing assistant applies direct pressure with his gloved hand.	_____
4. The nursing assistant encourages the patient to rest quietly after a seizure.	_____
5. After summoning help for the heart attack victim, the nursing assistant remains with the patient to offer emotional support.	_____

Moving Forward

Employment Opportunities and Career Growth

OBJECTIVES

After completing this unit, you will be able to:

- Spell and define terms.
- List nine objectives to be met in obtaining and maintaining employment.
- Follow a process for self-appraisal.
- Name sources of employment for nursing assistants.
- Prepare a résumé and a letter of resignation.
- List the steps for a successful interview.
- List the requirements that must be met when accepting employment.
- List steps for continuing development in your career.

UNIT SUMMARY

Finding the right employment after completion of your nursing assistant program can be easier if you set objectives and meet each one in a systematic fashion. The steps to take include:

- Appraising your assets and limitations.
- Searching the job market.

- Securing and holding the job.
- Properly resigning when it is time to make a career change.

Learning is a lifelong process. It may involve additional education and the ability to leave one position to move to another.

NURSING ASSISTANT ALERT

Action	Benefit
Be honest in your self-appraisals.	Provides accurate assessments upon which decisions can appropriately be made.
Conduct yourself in an ethical and proper manner.	Assures success in developing and maintaining successful employment opportunities.
Recognize that learning is a lifetime task.	Keeps your knowledge and skills updated.

ACTIVITIES

Vocabulary Exercise

Write the words forming the circle and define them.

1. _____

_____

2. _____

_____

3. _____

_____

4. _____

_____

Completion

Complete the following statements in the spaces provided.

1. One of the first steps in self-appraisal is to list all your _____ and _____.

2. It is important to think through possible _____ to any limitations to employment.

3. Preference for caring for a particular type of patient could influence your _____ options.

4. Home _____ and transportation are factors that might limit employment.

5. Talking with friends and colleagues about opportunities is called _____.

6 A written summary of work history is called a _____.

7. Always obtain _____ before giving a person's name as a reference.

8. Persons who are listed as references should know you well, but not be _____.

9. Clothing should be _____ and _____ for an interview.

10. It is important to be on _____ for an interview.

11. In a new work situation, there is much to learn from the examples of _____ staff workers.

12. When it is necessary to resign, do so in a _____ manner.

Short Answer

Briefly answer the following questions.

1. What will you specifically look for when seeking employment through classified ads?

   a. _____

   b. _____

   c. _____

   d. _____

2. What information should not be included in a résumé?

   a. _____

   b. _____

   c. _____

   d. _____

   e. _____

Practical Applications

Briefly describe the actions the nursing assistant might take in the following situations.

1. A classmate who is new to the area asks where nursing assistants can find employment in your community.

   _____

   _____

   _____

2. A family member asks what sources of information you will use as you begin your employment search.

   _____

   _____

3. Your teacher asks you to describe the practices you must keep in mind regarding a résumé.

   a. _____

   b. _____

   c. _____

   d. _____

   e. _____

   f. _____

4. List three things you will do when preparing for an interview.

a. _____

b. _____

c. _____

5. A classmate asks you to explain how you can make a new position more secure.

a. _____

b. _____

c. _____

d. _____

e. _____

6. A classmate asks you for six ways to enhance your knowledge and education after certification.

a. _____

b. _____

c. _____

d. _____

e. _____

f. _____

True/False

Mark the following true or false by circling T or F.

1. T F You should wait to be invited before sitting at an interview.

2. T F Body language is very important in conveying your interest in employment.

3. T F Ask for a job description to be sure you are qualified for the position being offered.

4. T F Mail your résumé after the interview.

5. T F Always thank the interviewer at the end of the interview.

6. T F View every interview as a learning experience, even if it doesn't go well.

7. T F Nursing and medical literature are good sources of information about patient conditions.

8. T F Always give a two-week notice before leaving a job.

9. T F Be positive in a resignation even if you are leaving a position because something upsetting has happened.

10. T F Always date and sign a letter of resignation.

Résumé Writing

1. Practice writing a résumé. When you have finished, check it against the list of areas to be covered.

a. your name, address, and telephone number

b. your educational background

c. your work history

d. other experiences you have had

e. references

f. personal information about interests and activities

Practice Résumé

2. Using your résumé, complete the employment application in the following figure.

GENERAL HOSPITAL
Application for Employment

1. Full Name: _____

      Last   First   Middle   Maiden

      _____

      Street and Number or Rural Route

      _____

      City, State and ZIP Code

      _____

      County   Telephone or nearest—Specify

      Social Security Number _____

2. Person to notify in case of emergency:
   Name _____
   Address _____

            _____
   Telephone _____
   Relationship _____

3. Education: List in this order—High School, College. You must give complete addresses. Also, please note if you did not graduate from high school whether or not you have a GED certificate.

School	Address	City	State	Year

4. Work or Vocational Experience: Give most recent first.

Name of Institution or Company	Complete Address	Type of Work	Dates

5. Have you ever been arrested for anything other than minor traffic violations? Yes ___ No ___
6. Are you now or have you been addicted to the use of alcohol or habit-forming drugs? Yes___ No___
7. References: Name three people who know your qualifications or who know your character. They must not be related to you.

   Name _____
   Address _____ Telephone _____

   Name _____
   Address _____ Telephone _____

   Name _____
   Address _____ Telephone _____

8. What are your reasons for wishing to work at this facility? Please answer this question in paragraph form on the back of this application.

3. In the following form, practice writing a letter of resignation by filling in the spaces provided.

           _____

                       (date)

Dear _____:

It is necessary for me to leave my position as _____

                                           (position)

as of _____. Working here at _____

          (effective date of resignation)   *(facility name)*

has given me an opportunity to _____.

I find I must leave because _____.

                                      (reason for leaving)

Thank you for your understanding of my situation.

                                 Sincerely,

                    _____

                                  (your name)

Student Performance Record

STUDENT PERFORMANCE RECORD

Your instructor will evaluate each procedure you learn and perform, but it will be helpful if you also keep a record so you will know which experiences you still must master.

PROCEDURE	Date	Satisfactory	Unsatisfactory
Unit 13 Infection Control			
Procedure 1 Handwashing			
Procedure 2 Putting on a Mask			
Procedure 3 Putting on a Gown			
Procedure 4 Putting on Gloves			
Procedure 5 Removing Contaminated Gloves			
Procedure 6 Removing Contaminated Gloves, Eye Protection, Gown, and Mask			
Procedure 7 Serving a Meal in an Isolation Unit			
Procedure 8 Measuring Vital Signs in an Isolation Unit			
Procedure 9 Transferring Nondisposable Equipment Outside of the Isolation Unit			
Procedure 10 Specimen Collection from a Patient in an Isolation Unit			
Procedure 11 Caring for Linens in an Isolation Unit			
Procedure 12 Transporting a Patient to and from the Isolation Unit			
Procedure 13 Opening a Sterile Package			
Unit 15 Patient Safety and Positioning			
Procedure 14 Turning the Patient Toward You			
Procedure 15 Turning the Patient Away from You			
Procedure 16 Moving a Patient to the Head of the Bed			
Procedure 17 Logrolling the Patient			
Unit 16 The Patient's Mobility: Transfer Skills			
Procedure 18 Applying a Transfer Belt			
Procedure 19 Transferring the Patient from Bed to Chair—One Assistant			
Procedure 20 Transferring the Patient from Bed to Chair—Two Assistants			
Procedure 21 Sliding-Board Transfer from Bed to Wheelchair			

PROCEDURE	Date	Satisfactory	Unsatisfactory
Procedure 22 Transferring the Patient from Chair to Bed—One Assistant			
Procedure 23 Transferring the Patient from Chair to Bed—Two Assistants			
Procedure 24 Independent Transfer, Standby Assist			
Procedure 25 Transferring the Patient from Bed to Stretcher			
Procedure 26 Transferring the Patient from Stretcher to Bed			
Procedure 27 Transferring the Patient with a Mechanical Lift			
Procedure 28 Transferring the Patient onto and off the Toilet			
Unit 17 The Patient's Mobility: Ambulation			
Procedure 29 Assisting the Patient to Walk with a Cane and Three-Point Gait			
Procedure 30 Assisting the Patient to Walk with a Walker and Three-Point Gait			
Procedure 31 Assisting the Falling Patient			
Unit 18 Body Temperature			
Procedure 32 Measuring an Oral Temperature (Electronic Thermometer)			
Procedure 33 Measuring a Rectal Temperature (Electronic Thermometer)			
Procedure 34 Measuring an Axillary Temperature (Electronic Thermometer)			
Procedure 35 Measuring a Tympanic Temperature			
Procedure 36 Measuring a Temporal Artery Temperature			
Unit 19 Pulse and Respiration			
Procedure 37 Counting the Radial Pulse			
Procedure 38 Counting the Apical-Radial Pulse			
Procedure 39 Counting Respirations			
Unit 20 Blood Pressure			
Procedure 40 Taking Blood Pressure			
Procedure 41 Taking Blood Pressure with an Electronic Blood Pressure Apparatus			

PROCEDURE	Date	Satisfactory	Unsatisfactory
Unit 21 Measuring Height and Weight			
Procedure 42 Weighing and Measuring the Patient Using an Upright Scale			
Procedure 43 Weighing the Patient on a Chair Scale			
Procedure 44 Measuring Weight with an Electronic Wheelchair Scale			
Procedure 45 Measuring and Weighing the Patient in Bed			
Unit 22 Admission, Transfer, and Discharge			
Procedure 46 Admitting the Patient			
Procedure 47 Transferring the Patient			
Procedure 48 Discharging the Patient			
Unit 23 Bedmaking			
Procedure 49 Making a Closed Bed			
Procedure 50 Opening the Closed Bed			
Procedure 51 Making an Occupied Bed			
Procedure 52 Making the Surgical Bed			
Unit 24 Patient Bathing			
Procedure 53 Assisting with the Tub Bath or Shower			
Procedure 54 Bed Bath			
Procedure 55 Changing the Patient's Gown			
Procedure 56 Waterless Bed Bath			
Procedure 57 Partial Bath			
Procedure 58 Female Perineal Care			
Procedure 59 Male Perineal Care			
Procedure 60 Hand and Fingernail Care			
Procedure 61 Bed Shampoo			
Procedure 62 Dressing and Undressing the Patient			
Unit 25 General Comfort Measures			
Procedure 63 Assisting with Routine Oral Hygiene			
Procedure 64 Assisting with Special Oral Hygiene—Dependent and Unconscious Patients			
Procedure 65 Assisting the Patient to Floss and Brush Teeth			
Procedure 66 Caring for Dentures			

PROCEDURE	Date	Satisfactory	Unsatisfactory
Procedure 67 Backrub			
Procedure 68 Shaving a Male Patient			
Procedure 69 Daily Hair Care			
Procedure 70 Giving and Receiving the Bedpan			
Procedure 71 Giving and Receiving the Urinal			
Procedure 72 Assisting with Use of the Bedside Commode			
Unit 26 Nutritional Needs and Diet Modifications			
Procedure 73 Assisting the Patient Who Can Feed Self			
Procedure 74 Feeding the Dependent Patient			
Procedure 75 Abdominal Thrusts—Heimlich Maneuver			
Unit 27 Warm and Cold Applications			
Procedure 76 Applying an Ice Bag or Gel Pack			
Procedure 77 Applying a Disposable Cold Pack			
Procedure 78 Applying an Aquamatic K-Pad			
Procedure 79 Giving a Sitz Bath			
Procedure 80 Assisting with Application of an Aquathermia Blanket			
Unit 29 The Surgical Patient			
Procedure 81 Assisting the Patient to Deep Breathe and Cough			
Procedure 82 Performing Postoperative Leg Exercises			
Procedure 83 Applying Elasticized Stockings			
Procedure 84 Applying an Elastic Bandage			
Procedure 85 Applying Pneumatic Compression Hosiery			
Procedure 86 Assisting the Patient to Dangle			
Unit 32 Death and Dying			
Procedure 87 Giving Postmortem Care			
Unit 36 Subacute Care			
Procedure 88 Setting Up a Sterile Field Using a Sterile Drape			
Procedure 89 Adding an Item to a Sterile Field			
Procedure 90 Adding Liquids to a Sterile Field			
Procedure 91 Applying and Removing Sterile Gloves			

PROCEDURE	Date	Satisfactory	Unsatisfactory
Procedure 92 Using Transfer Forceps			
Procedure 93 Applying a Dry Sterile Dressing			
Procedure 94 Discontinuing a Peripheral IV			
Procedure 95 Applying a Dressing Around a Drain			
Procedure 96 Care of a T-Tube or Similar Wound Drain			
Procedure 97 Removing Sutures			
Procedure 98 Removing Staples			
Unit 38 Integumentary System			
Procedure 99 Changing a Clean Dressing and Applying a Bandage			
Procedure 100 Applying a Transparent Film Dressing			
Procedure 101 Applying a Hydrocolloid Dressing			
Unit 39 Respiratory System			
Procedure 102 Checking Capillary Refill			
Procedure 103 Using a Pulse Oximeter			
Procedure 104 Collecting a Sputum Specimen			
Unit 41 Musculoskeletal System			
Procedure 105 Assisting with Continuous Passive Motion			
Procedure 106 Performing Range-of-Motion Exercises (Passive)			
Unit 42 Endocrine System			
Procedure 107 Obtaining a Fingerstick Blood Sugar			
Unit 43 Nervous System			
Procedure 108 Caring for the Eye Socket and Artificial Eye			
Procedure 109 Applying Warm or Cool Eye Compresses			
Unit 44 Gastrointestinal System			
Procedure 110 Collecting a Stool Specimen			
Procedure 111 Testing for Occult Blood Using Hemoccult and Developer			
Procedure 112 Inserting a Rectal Suppository			
Procedure 113 Giving a Soap-Solution Enema			
Procedure 114 Giving a Commercially Prepared Enema			

PROCEDURE	Date	Satisfactory	Unsatisfactory
Procedure 115 Inserting a Rectal Tube and Flatus Bag			
Procedure 116 Giving Routine Stoma Care (Colostomy)			
Procedure 117 Routine Care of an Ileostomy (with Patient in Bed)			
Unit 45 Urinary System			
Procedure 118 Collecting a Routine Urine Specimen			
Procedure 119 Collecting a Clean-Catch Urine Specimen			
Procedure 120 Collecting a 24-Hour Urine Specimen			
Procedure 121 Collecting a Urine Specimen Through a Drainage Port			
Procedure 122 Routine Drainage Check			
Procedure 123 Giving Indwelling Catheter Care			
Procedure 124 Emptying a Urinary Drainage Unit			
Procedure 125 Disconnecting the Catheter			
Procedure 126 Applying a Condom for Urinary Drainage			
Procedure 127 Connecting a Catheter to a Leg Bag			
Procedure 128 Emptying a Leg Bag			
Procedure 129 Removing an Indwelling Catheter			
Unit 46 Reproductive System			
Procedure 130 Giving a Nonsterile Vaginal Douche			
Unit 49 Obstetrical Patients and Neonates			
Procedure 131 Changing a Diaper			
Procedure 132 Weighing the Infant			
Procedure 133 Measuring the Infant			
Procedure 134 Bathing an Infant			
Procedure 135 Bottle-Feeding an Infant			
Procedure 136 Assisting with Breastfeeding			
Procedure 137 Burping an Infant			
Unit 50 Pediatric Patients			
Procedure 138 Admitting a Pediatric Patient			
Procedure 139 Weighing the Toddler to Adolescent			
Procedure 140 Changing Crib Linens			
Procedure 141 Changing Crib Linens (Infant in Crib)			

PROCEDURE	Date	Satisfactory	Unsatisfactory
Procedure 142 Measuring Temperature			
Procedure 143 Determining Heart Rate (Pulse)			
Procedure 144 Counting Respiratory Rate			
Procedure 145 Measuring Blood Pressure			
Procedure 146 Collecting a Urine Specimen from an Infant			
Unit 51 Response to Basic Emergencies			
Procedure 147 Head-Tilt, Chin-Lift Maneuver			
Procedure 148 Jaw-Thrust Maneuver			
Procedure 149 Mask-to-Mouth Ventilation			
Procedure 150 Positioning the Patient in the Recovery Position			
Procedure 151 Assisting the Adult Who Has an Obstructed Airway and Becomes Unconscious			
Procedure 152 Obstructed Airway: Infant			
Procedure 153 Child with Foreign Body Airway Obstruction			

PART 3

Nursing Assistant Written State Test Overview

VOCABULARY

standardized testing	taking the test
state test content	miscellaneous testing concerns
taking a multiple-choice test	the skills examination
study skills	after the test

STANDARDIZED TESTING

The state certification test you will be taking is a **standardized test**. This means it was written so that it will be fair to everyone who takes the test. A test becomes standardized only after having been piloted, used, revised, and used again until it shows consistent results. The purpose of a standardized test is to establish an average score, or *norm*. This allows one person's scores to be compared with the scores of many others across the state or country. A standardized test must be given in the same way each time. This is done by using the same plan and the same directions. The examiner is allowed to give only certain kinds of help. The conditions at all test sites should be similar, and each answer is scored according to definite rules.

The written state test is designed to ensure that you have the knowledge necessary to function safely as an entry-level (beginning) nursing assistant. The test varies in each state. For most states, the test has between 50 and 120 questions. You will be given approximately 2 hours to complete the written test, depending on length. The test may include approximately 10 extra questions that are not scored. These are in the process of being standardized for use in future tests. You will not know which questions are scored and which are unscored. The time allowed for completing the test is fairly generous. The test examiner will call time near the end of the test to warn you that the end of the allotted time is near.

The written test questions are all in multiple-choice format. Although some questions are difficult, there are no trick questions. Questions are developed by experienced nursing assistant educators and are designed to measure the competency of an average learner. They are not designed to punish slow learners or reward faster learners. Various terms may be used to describe the person giving care. For testing purposes, the term *nurse aide* is commonly used to describe the caregiver, but other terms, such as *nurse assistant* and *nursing assistant*, may be used in your state. The word *client* is commonly used to describe the person receiving care, but the terms *patient* and *resident* may also be used. Your examiner will inform you of the proper terms for these individuals. The questions on the test will be arranged randomly and will not be grouped together by specific category or subject.

Many states have a practice test and candidate handbook available. Ask your instructor if these tools are available in your state. They will be extremely valuable in preparing for your state test. Many practice state tests are online at http://www.promissor.com/, http://www.respondus.com/, and http://www.prometric.com/. Some state nursing assistant registries also maintain websites. If your state registry is online, you may wish to check its website for information about the state test.

STATE TEST CONTENT

The National Nurse Aide Assessment Program (NNAAP) forms the basis for the examination questions. The purpose of the NNAAP Written (or Oral) Examination is to make sure that you understand the responsibilities and can safely perform the job duties of an entry-level nursing assistant. The OBRA law of 1987 was designed to improve the quality of care in long-term care facilities and to establish training and examination standards for nursing assistants. Each state is responsible for following the terms of this federal law. The examination is a measure of knowledge, skills, and abilities related to nursing assisting. There are two parts to the examination: written and skills. Both parts are usually given on the same day.

The nursing assistant state written test covers the main content areas that you studied in class. These are:

Physical Care Skills

- Activities of daily living (ADLs)/Promotion of health and safety

  ◦ Hygiene

  ◦ Dressing and grooming

  ◦ Nutrition and hydration

  ◦ Elimination

  ◦ Comfort, rest, and sleep

Basic Nursing Skills

- Infection control

- Safety and emergency procedures

- Therapeutic and technical procedures, such as bedmaking, specimen collection, measurement of height and weight, and use of restraints

- Observation, reporting, and data collection

Restorative Nursing Care Skills/Promotion of Function and Health

- Preventive health care, such as contracture and pressure ulcer prevention

- Promotion of client self-care and independence

Psychosocial Care Skills/Specialized Care

- Emotional and mental health needs

  ◦ Behavior management

  ◦ Needs of the dying client

  ◦ Sexuality needs

  ◦ Cultural and spiritual needs

Roles and Responsibilities of the Nursing Assistant

- Communication

  ◦ Verbal communication

  ◦ Nonverbal communication

  ◦ Listening

  ◦ Clients with special communication problems

- Resident rights (long-term care)

- Legal and ethical behavior

- Responsibilities as a member of the health care team

- Knowledge of medical terminology and abbreviations

TAKING A MULTIPLE-CHOICE TEST

Most standardized tests use multiple-choice items. This is because multiple-choice items can measure a variety of learning outcomes, from simple to complex. They also provide the most consistent results. Each multiple-choice item consists of a **stem**, which presents a problem situation, and four possible choices called **alternatives**. The alternatives include the correct answer and several wrong answers called **distractors**. The stem may be a question or incomplete statement as shown:

Question form:

Q. Which of the following people is responsible for taking care of a client?

    a. janitor

    b. administrator

    c. nursing assistant

    d. social worker

Incomplete statement form:

Q. The care of a client is the responsibility of a:

    a. janitor

    b. administrator

    c. nursing assistant

    d. social worker

Although worded differently, both stems present the same problem. The alternatives in the examples contain only one correct answer. All distractors are clearly incorrect.

Another type of multiple-choice item is the best-answer format. In this format, the alternatives *may be partially correct*, but one is clearly better than the others. Look at the following example:

Best-answer form:

Q. Which of the following ethical behaviors is the MOST important?

    a. Maintain a positive attitude.

    b. Act as a responsible employee.

    c. Be courteous to visitors.

    d. Promote quality of life for each client.

Other variations of the best-answer form may ask you, "What is the first thing to do," what is the "most helpful action," what is the "best response" or "best answer," or a similar kind of question. Whether the correct-answer form or best-answer form is used depends on the information given.

Each multiple-choice question lists four answers. The chance of guessing correctly is only one in four, or 25%. Each test question has only one correct answer. Do not mark more than one answer per item, or the item will be marked wrong. Do not leave answers blank.

STUDY SKILLS

No matter what type of test you take, you must first master the material. Using index cards is an excellent way to do this. You may wish to prepare index cards listing vocabulary terms, abbreviations, or questions from your workbook or text. Using index cards to create study or flashcards will enable you to test your ability to recognize and retrieve important information.

To study, read the front of the card and try to answer the question. Turn the card over to see if you are correct. After going through all the cards once, you may wish to shuffle them and review them again. Make sure you know the information and can answer questions in any order.

As you review the cards, begin to sort them into two piles. One pile is for those you know well; the other pile is for those you are having trouble remembering. Once you have two piles, try to learn the most difficult information. Continue reviewing the cards until you have mastered the material. Review the cards several times a day during the time before the exam.

There are several advantages to using the card system. First, sorting the cards and preparing extra cards is a good learning experience. Second, the cards are easy and convenient to carry with you in a purse or pocket. You can study them during spare moments throughout the day. Another advantage is that you can use the cards with a friend to quiz each other.

Other Helpful Study Skills

1. Block out a specific time for study. Study your biorhythms to find the time of day when you are functioning at your peak level of performance.

2. Get plenty of sleep.

3. Begin studying well before the state certification test. Schedule your study sessions so that you can take a break in between. For example, studying for an hour in the morning and an hour in the evening is more effective than studying for two consecutive hours. Trying to study when you are mentally or physically tired is a waste of time.

4. Study the most difficult material when you are most alert.

5. Control your environment. Do whatever it takes to find a quiet place to study. Get up early in the morning, when everyone else is asleep, or find a quiet corner of the library.

6. Become part of a small, dedicated study group of three to five people, or find a study partner.

7. Eat a healthful diet, especially protein and complex carbohydrates.

8. Study key concepts by asking yourself, "What are four different ways this idea could be tested?"

9. Learn the rationale behind each issue. Write a brief statement of rationale on the back of each index card with the answer. Study all of the information included in the rationale on your study cards. Ask yourself how the information could be tested. Make sure you can apply the principles and rationale to similar situations.

10. You may also create study checklists. Identify all the material for which you are accountable. Break it down into manageably sized lists of steps, notes, and procedures for each item. For example, write down the steps of a nursing procedure. Create a separate column for supplies needed and any special information you need to know.

11. Record your notes or study questions on audiotape or other recording device such as your smartphone. You may play the recording at home or in the car when you are commuting.

12. Many excellent tools and resources for studying are available online at http://www.studygs.net/

Stress and Test Anxiety

You may be surprised to learn that stress is normal. A certain amount of stress can be good. Almost everyone has some test anxiety. Studies have shown that mild stress actually improves performance by athletes, entertainers, public speakers, and test takers! "Butterflies" in the stomach, breathing faster, sweating, and other symptoms are automatic body responses to stressful situations. Stress can sharpen your attention, keep you alert, and give you greater energy. Remember, it is not the stress that is harmful, but your reaction to it. Learn and practice how to control stress. Some stress cannot be avoided, but you will know the date of this exam well in advance. Try to avoid other stressful situations immediately before the test. Prepare yourself physically and mentally.

If you feel stressed immediately before or during the exam, try a deep-breathing activity recommended by stress management experts. Breathe slowly and deeply from the diaphragm. Do not move the chest and shoulders. You should feel your abdominal muscles expand when you inhale and relax when you exhale. As you breathe out, your diaphragm and rib muscles seem to relax and your body may seem to sink down into the chair. This helps promote relaxation. Sixty seconds of controlled deep breathing helps relieve stress.

Factors that increase stress and test anxiety are negative thoughts and self-doubt. Perhaps you have thought, "I am going to fail this exam. What will my family or coworkers think if I do not pass?" You must control your reaction to this stress and stop thinking these thoughts. Instead, say to yourself, "I have done this job successfully. I know this material, and did well in class. I am going to pass this examination." View the exam as an opportunity to show what you know and can do. Positive thinking comes before positive action and positive results. Consciously stop negative thoughts and force them out by using positive ones instead.

TAKING THE TEST

To do well on a test, you should be at your best when you start. Eat a good breakfast or lunch. Try to avoid anything that will cause stress. Dress appropriately, according to exam center requirements. Candidates who are not properly attired may be denied admission.

Be on time. If you are late, you may not be admitted. If you miss the test, your testing fees may not be refundable, and you will lose your money. If weather conditions are unsafe, the test may be canceled and rescheduled. If you are absent because of a valid emergency, you must promptly submit proof of this emergency to the testing service (usually within 30 days). Examples of acceptable excuses are a death in the immediate family, disabling traffic accident, illness of yourself or an immediate family member, jury duty, court appearance, or military duty. A service fee may be charged if you miss the test, even if you have proof of an acceptable excuse.

Leave for the test site early enough to arrive on time. Allow a little extra time for minor delays. In some states, you may be required to arrive up to 30 minutes early to allow time for registration, processing, verification of identification, and sign-in.

Take a watch and several (two or three) number 2, sharpened black lead pencils with erasers. If your state issues an admission letter, bring it with you and present it to the examiner. Most states have a list of supplies or identification that you must bring to be admitted to the test. Most require a photo identification, and some require you to produce your original social security card, or to furnish a copy of that card. Your photo identification should be a government-issued document, such as a driver's license, state identification card, or passport. The name on the photo identification should be the same as the name used to register for the test, including suffixes such as "Jr.," "III," and the like. The photo identification card must also bear your signature. Each state has a list of acceptable identification that is given to candidates when they register for the test. If you do not have proper photo identification, contact the testing service well in advance to make arrangements for using an alternate means of identification. Some states require two different forms of identification. Learn the requirements in advance and be prepared to meet them. In addition, some states require fingerprinting by a law enforcement agency prior to testing. It is the applicant's responsibility to see that this has been done in a timely manner, and to pay all associated fees. You may be required to bring the official (completed) fingerprint card with you at the time of testing. If you are late or fail to bring the required identification or supplies, you may not be admitted, so follow directions carefully.

You will not be permitted to bring audio or video recording devices or personal communication devices, such as pagers and cell phones, into the test site. Likewise, you may not bring children, visitors, or pets. (Service animals are not considered pets and will be admitted.) Do not bring valuables or weapons. You probably will not be permitted to bring personal items other than your keys into the exam room. Leave purses, backpacks, books, notes, and other items in the car. You will not be permitted to eat, drink, or smoke during the examination. Students who display disruptive behavior will be removed and their exam scores recorded as a failure. If necessary, the skills examiner will call law enforcement authorities to remove or manage a disruptive candidate.

When you arrive at the test site, do not let another person's last-minute questions or comments upset you. Do not talk about the test with other students, if possible. Anxiety is contagious. Follow these general rules for taking the test:

1. Choose a good spot to sit. Make sure you have enough space. Maintain good posture and do not slouch. Be comfortable but alert. Stay relaxed and confident.

2. Remind yourself that you are well prepared and are going to do well. If you become anxious, take several slow, deep breaths to relax.

3. You will be given verbal instructions and be asked to complete an information form. Pay close attention to the examiner's instructions. He or she will read the directions. The examiner may not be permitted to answer questions.

4. Take several more deep breaths and try to relax. If you become anxious during the test, close your eyes for a few seconds and practice slow, deep breathing. Remaining relaxed and positive are keys to success. Remind yourself that you have studied well and are prepared to take the test. Think positive.

5. When you receive your test booklet, review the written directions and look at any sample questions. Make sure you understand how to mark your answers. Follow directions carefully. Most state tests are scored by computer, and stray marks may cause otherwise correct answers to be marked wrong. Write only on your answer sheet. Answers written in the exam book will not be counted.

6. Work at a steady pace.

7. Take the questions at face value. Do not read anything into them. Avoid thinking, "what if?" Answer the question based on the information given. Do not look for trick questions or hidden meanings. Do not add or subtract information.

8. Read the stem of the question. Think of the answer in your own words before reading the answers. Then read all of the answers given. Search for the correct alternative, then select the option that most closely matches your answer. If necessary, read the stem with each option. If you are still not sure, treat each option as a true-false question, and choose the "most true."

9. It may be helpful to cross out unnecessary words in the question. Distracting information has been crossed out in this example:

   Q. A client ~~who~~ is HIV positive ~~understands that the nurse aide will not talk about this information outside the facility because~~ this information is:

   a. legal.

   b. confidential.

   c. negligent.

   d. cultural.

10. If you do not know the answer to a question, circle the number and move on. Come back to it later. You may remember the answer later, or may find a clue to the answer in another question. Do not waste time struggling with questions you are unsure of. This increases your stress and test anxiety. Continuing with the test is best.

11. Be alert to words such as *not* and *except* that may completely change the intent of the question. Pay close attention to words that are *italicized*, CAPITALIZED, or are within "quotation marks" or (parentheses). Words such as *first, last, most, least, best,* and *except* often hold the key to the answer. Read carefully. These words are usually very important.

12. Avoid unfamiliar choices. Information that you are unfamiliar with is probably incorrect.

13. If you do not know the answer, try to identify answers that are not correct. Cross out answers that you know or think are incorrect. If you have crossed out two answers, you have a 50% chance of guessing correctly. Other suggestions for eliminating incorrect answers are to cross out:

   a. Question options that grammatically do not fit with the stem

   b. Question options that are completely unfamiliar to you

   c. Question options that contain negative or absolute words, such as those listed in number 11 above.

Some other strategies may also be useful:

a. Substitute a qualified term for the absolute one, such as "frequently" instead of "always." This may help you eliminate another incorrect answer.

b. If two answers seem correct, compare them for differences, then refer to the stem to find your best answer.

c. Use hints from questions you know to help you answer questions that you are not sure of.

14. Look at the shortest and longest of the remaining answers. The correct answer may be shorter or longer than the others.

15. There is no penalty for guessing. If you cannot figure out the answer, guessing is better than leaving a question blank.

16. Do not become upset or nervous if some individuals finish the test early and get up to leave. Some people read faster than others. Studies have shown that those who finish first do not necessarily get the best scores.

17. When you get to the end of the test, go back and complete the items you skipped.

18. Do not change your answers without a good reason. Your first answer is more likely to be correct. Change the answer if you misread or misunderstood the question, or if you are absolutely certain the first answer is wrong.

19. Before turning the test in, check it to make sure you marked every answer. Check the circles or boxes to be sure they are completely marked on the computer scoring sheet. Erase all stray marks.

MISCELLANEOUS TESTING CONCERNS

- In some states, the written test is given on a computer. If you are taking a computerized test, you will be given several practice questions to make sure you know how to use the computer. Complete the practice questions. If you have difficulty in using the computer, speak with the skills examiner.

- Most states administer oral examinations if special circumstances exist. Some states give examinations in languages other than English. These special examinations must be requested from your state testing agency when you register to take the test. If you think you need an oral examination or non-English version of the test, contact your instructor or state testing service for information and instructions. The oral examinations are typically recorded. You will listen to the recording with a headset. Typically, each question is read twice in a neutral manner. You will also be furnished with a written test booklet so you can review the printed words while listening to the tape. You will answer the question by marking in the answer sheet. However, to be a nursing assistant, you must be able to read and write in English. Even if you take an oral or non-English examination, you will be given a series of reading comprehension questions, typically 10. You must pass this portion of the examination, showing your understanding of the English language, in order to pass the exam as a whole. The time limits for oral testing are usually the same as the time limits for the written test.

- Your state will accommodate individuals with certain disabilities during the test. Contact your state testing agency well in advance for information on requesting accommodations. You cannot wait until the day of the test to request a special accommodation.

- Your state will have a skills (manual competency) examination portion of the state certification test. You must pass both portions of the test before being entered into the nursing assistant registry. Contact your instructor or state testing agency for information.

- *Do not bring personal communication devices, such as pagers, telephones, tablets, or other electronic devices, to the test site.* Use of these items is not permitted, and you will not be allowed to take them into the test site.

Test Security

- Do not give help to anyone or receive help from anyone during the test. If the examiner suspects a candidate of cheating on the examination, he or she will end that candidate's test and ask the individual to leave. The score will be recorded as a failure. The examiner reports individuals who cheat on the test to the state nursing assistant registry.

- When you have finished testing, turn all paper materials in. You may not remove the examination booklet, notes, or papers from the room.

- Individuals caught removing a test from the testing site may be prosecuted. Copying, displaying, or distributing a copyrighted examination is illegal.

The Skills Examination

Part of the state test is a skills examination. This examination is administered slightly differently in each state. Usually, a nurse who has no affiliation with your school or educational program administers the examination. You will be tested on the number of skills required by your state. Your skills will be chosen at random from the required skills list for your state. In most states, five skills are tested.

Reporting to the nurse, documenting, and doing basic calculations are parts of some skills. For example, if you weigh a patient, you must calculate the total value from the upper and lower bars of the scale correctly. If you take a rectal or axillary temperature, you must show the skills examiner that you know how to record it correctly by placing an "R" or "A" after the temperature reading. If you count the pulse or respirations for 30 seconds, you must calculate and document the full-minute value correctly. If a value is abnormal, such as a temperature of 103.6°F (R), you must recognize that the value is abnormal and report it to the nurse or proper person. (In this case, inform the skills examiner of the abnormal value and state that you would report it to the nurse. If you are taking the test on a real patient, notify the nurse promptly as soon as the exam has ended, or ask the examiner's permission to leave briefly to report.) If you empty a catheter bag or measure intake and output, you must use a graduate, measure, calculate, add, and document the total(s) correctly. This also applies to estimating meal intake and other measurements and calculations on the examination. If you are concerned about your math skills, ask your instructor if you will be permitted to use a calculator. If so, take one with you to the exam.

The passing rate for the skills component of the exam will vary with your state. Commonly, you must pass four or five skills to pass the examination. However, you do not have to complete each skill perfectly. Certain steps are designated as critical points in the skill. If you perform these correctly, you will pass the skill, even if you make a mistake. In some states, this testing is done in the skills laboratory using other students as patient volunteers. The examiner reads the student volunteer a statement and gives instructions on what is expected in playing the role of the patient. Treat the student volunteer exactly as you would a patient. Some skills, such as perineal care, may be done on a manikin. Pretend the manikin is a patient, and treat it with the same courtesy and precautions as you would use for a patient. All equipment and supplies will be available to perform the skill, but you must know what you need and gather it before beginning. Ask questions before you begin testing on the skill. Once the test begins, the nurse examiner will be unable to answer questions.

Some states do the state skills test only on residents in a nursing facility. Some states time the skills examination. For example, you may be given 35 minutes in which to complete this portion of the test. Some states require you to pass the written test first, before you will be permitted to take the skills exam. In other states, the opposite is true: You must pass the skills examination before you will be permitted to take the written test. Although foreign-language options are available for the written test, the skills examination is given only in English.

Preparing for the Skills Examination

The only way to adequately prepare for the skills examination is to practice each procedure in sequence. If you practice, the skills will become automatic. The skills that you will be tested on are randomly selected from the procedures you learned in class. If your nursing assistant class has a review day or mock skills examination before you take the test, be sure to attend. This will be very helpful to you in preparing for the test.

You should also review your vocabulary terms so you are familiar with the various names for the procedures. For example, the skills examiner may direct you to "ambulate the patient." From your review of the vocabulary, you know that *ambulate* means to walk. If the examiner instructs you to do range-of-motion exercises on the lower *extremities*, you must know that these are the *legs*. Practice your skills with other students or with your family, and use your procedure checklists or forms provided by your state.

When reviewing the procedures, pay close attention to the list of supplies and equipment you will need to gather before you perform the procedure. It is essential that you collect the right supplies at the time of the skills test, or you may be unable to complete a procedure.

There is no way to study for the skills examination other than reviewing and practicing the procedures you learned in class. The skills examiner will watch for certain things during the examination. Some of these observations are very important and may be the deciding factor on whether you pass or fail a particular skill on the examination.

Observations Made During the Skills Examination

Gather all the supplies you will need before beginning each section of the test. If you will be making the bed, stack the linen in order of use. The test will go more smoothly if you are well organized.

Direct Care

Most of the skills examination consists of **direct care activities**. Direct patient care activities assist patients in meeting basic human needs, such as feeding, drinking, positioning, ambulating, grooming, toileting, and dressing. They may involve collecting, recording, and reporting information.

Indirect Care

Certain skills are part of every procedure that you perform. These are usually called **indirect care skills**. Indirect activities focus on maintaining the environment and the systems in which nursing care is delivered. They assist in providing a clean, efficient, safe, comfortable, respectful patient care environment. An indirect care skill is an important part of the procedure, but does not necessarily affect the outcome. Data collection, documentation, consultation with other health care providers, and reporting of information are indirect care skills. Examples of indirect care tasks are communication, comfort, patient rights, safety, and infection control. The skills examiner will look closely at (and score) your indirect care skills in each and every procedure. Doing these things each and every time is critical to your success. Indirect care skills on which you will be tested include the following essential elements:

- The skills examiner will observe **handwashing**. He or she will monitor your handwashing technique to be sure that you follow accepted standards and procedures. Wash your hands before and after caring for each patient, and more often as necessary. This skill will not be prompted by the examiner, meaning that you will not be told or reminded to do it. Nursing assistants are expected to know when and how to wash their hands. Use the proper technique. Each handwashing should last a minimum of 15–20 seconds, or according to your state rules. You may be permitted to use alcohol-based hand cleaner unless your hands are soiled. Consult your instructor on this in advance. However, the skills examiner may still request you to do at least one handwash at the sink so that he or she can see whether you have mastered the skill.

- **Infection control** is another area on which you are evaluated. The skills examiner observes your technique in patient care, the use of standard precautions and medical asepsis. The examiner will also observe if you wear gloves and other personal protective equipment (PPE) when necessary. You will be evaluated on whether you wash your hands before applying and removing gloves, as well as using proper technique in applying and removing the gloves themselves. Other important considerations are keeping clean and soiled items separated, disposing of soiled articles correctly, and preventing environmental contamination from used gloves and equipment.

- The examiner will observe how well you **communicate** with each patient. You must introduce yourself and the skills examiner. Explain what you are going to do, even if the patient is confused. Inform the patient before each step, such as "Now I am going to turn you over on your side." You may also be evaluated on whether you speak with the person throughout the procedure.

- The skills examiner will observe how well you practice **safety**. In fact, many safety violations constitute automatic test failures, such as leaving the bedside with the bed in the high position and side rails down. Another example is failure to lock the wheelchair brakes before transferring the patient. These are potentially serious problems that could result in patient injuries, so the skills examiners take them very seriously. Protect patient safety throughout the procedure. When you have finished the procedure, make sure the patient is left safe, with the call signal within reach. Do not leave the room if the patient is in an unsafe location or position, or if the ordered side rails or restraints are not in place.

- Protecting and honoring **patient rights** is also very important. Be sure to knock on doors and wait for permission to enter. Use the bath blanket for modesty when the patient's body will be exposed, such as during bathing and perineal care. Pull the privacy curtain, close the window curtains, and close the door to the room. Speak with the patient in a dignified manner. Avoid terms such as "honey," "dear," "granny," and "sweetie." Although facility staff may call patients by endearing names, the skills examiner will consider it undignified and unprofessional. Treat patients with the utmost respect. The nurse examiner will monitor your attention to the patient's dignity, privacy, and safety.

- Patient **comfort** is an important consideration. You must ensure patients' comfort by doing things such as handling patients gently, asking about their comfort, supporting the arm when taking blood pressure, positioning patients in good body alignment, and leaving each patient in a comfortable position upon completion of the skill.

Critical Points

Critical points are things that could potentially harm a patient. If you skip a critical point on your state skills examination, you will fail the skill. If your state or program uses skills checklists with key or critical points listed, pay close attention to them. For example, in many states, failure to balance the scale before weighing a patient is a critical (automatic failure) point.

Studying the critical points for each skill will be very helpful to you. Because these things could potentially harm a patient, you will feel more confident in providing care on the nursing units. Learning the critical points for each skill creates a win-win situation for both you and the patients. The following is an example of an actual skills test from one state. The underlined steps are the critical skills or automatic failure points.

Handwashing

1. Turns on water.
2. Wets hands.
3. Applies skin cleanser or soap to hands.
4. Rubs hands together for at least 15–20 seconds in a circular motion.
5. Washes all surfaces of the hands at least up to the wrist.
6. Rinses hands thoroughly from wrist to fingertips; cleans under fingernails, if needed, fingers down, under running water.
7. Dries hands on clean paper towel/warm air dryer.
8. Turns off faucet with paper towel and/or avoids contact with sink or other dirty surfaces during rinsing and drying of the hands.
9. Discards wet towel appropriately.

When taking the skills test, think through each task that is asked of you. If the nurse examiner tells you that your patient has had a stroke with right-side paralysis, and then instructs you to get the patient out of bed, think about which side the patient will transfer to, where you will position the wheelchair, how you will keep the patient safe, and whether another assistant is needed to help. Critical points for this skill will include locking the wheelchair brakes and using a transfer belt (unless contraindicated).

Other Mistakes

If you think you have made a mistake or forgot to do something during the skills examination, inform the skills examiner immediately. He or she may allow you to go back and correct the problem. This depends on the nature of the error and when you notify the examiner. If you inform the examiner of the error in a timely manner, he or she may permit you to go back and begin again at the point where the error was made. The skills examiner will not correct you if you make an error. He or she will not answer questions about the procedure during the test. If you have questions, ask them before testing begins. The skills examiner will not assist you or intervene during the test unless an unsafe patient condition develops.

AFTER THE TEST

After the test, you will breathe a sigh of relief. Listen carefully to the examiner's instructions for returning test materials. Information may also be provided about how and when you will find out the test results. In many states, you get preliminary results the same day. You will not be given a percentage or letter grade. Preliminary scores are listed as either "pass" or "fail." The results are considered preliminary until they are validated by the testing agency in its offices. After the tests are validated, you will be given a more complete explanation of your score. You should receive a report in the mail in approximately two weeks. If you have not received the results within 30 days, contact the examination service.

If you have passed the written and skills examinations, your name will be entered into your state nursing assistant registry. This may take several weeks. In some states, the criminal background and fingerprint checks must also be completed and cleared before you are entered into the registry.

In some states, the nurse examiner will fax your answer sheet for scoring as soon as you finish the exam. You will receive an official score report before leaving the test center. The report will indicate whether you have passed or failed the written (or oral) exam.

You will be issued a wallet card to show as proof of your certification. Protect your wallet card and do not lose it. Never give your employer or a prospective employer the original. If someone needs a copy, make a photocopy and keep the original in a safe place. If you lose your card, your state will issue a duplicate, but there is usually a fee for this service. Your certification must be current for the state to issue a duplicate card. Do not alter your card in any way. Altering the card may result in loss of certification.

The test is fair and most candidates pass the first time. If you did not pass the test, you will have at least two more opportunities to retest. You have three opportunities to pass each part of the examination. However, there is a fee for each retesting. Your instructor may have to register you for the retest. All testing fees must be submitted to the testing service at the time of registration. Meet with your instructor to find out what to study to increase your chances of successfully passing the retest.

You must keep your state nursing assistant registry informed of any changes in your name or address. If you move or change your name, notify the state registry promptly in writing. Provide your state registration number or social security number so the information can be listed for the proper person. (More than one person may have the same name.) Many states have forms for change of name or address available on their websites.

Your nursing assistant certification will expire in 24 months. To renew it, you must meet your state continuing education requirements. To remain active, you must submit a form verifying that you have provided paid nursing assistant services during the renewal period. The number of hours you are required to work to maintain your certification varies with each state.

Flashcards

abdomin/o	cephal/o
aden/o	cerebr/o
adren/o	chol/e
angi/o	chondr/o
arteri/o	col/o
arthr/o	cost/o
bronch/o	crani/o
card, cardi/o	cyst/o

head	abdomen
brain	gland
bile	adrenal gland
cartilage	vessel
colon, large intestine	artery
rib	joint
skull	bronchus, bronchi
bladder, cyst	heart

cyt/o	gloss/o
dent/o	hem, hema
derma	hemo, hemat
encephal/o	hepat/o
enter/o	hyster/o
erythr/o	ile/o
gastr/o	lapar/o
geront/o	laryng/o

tongue	cell
blood	tooth
blood	skin
liver	brain
uterus	small intestine
ileum	red
abdomen, loin, flank	stomach
larynx	old age

mamm/o	oophor/o
mast/o	ophthalm/o
men/o	oste/o
my/o	ot/o
myel/o	pharyng/o
nephr/o	phleb/o
neur/o	pneum/o
ocul/o	proct/o

ovary	breast
eye	breast
bone	menstruation
ear	muscle
pharynx	spinal cord, bone marrow
vein	kidney
lung, air, gas	nerve
rectum	eye

psych/o	thorac/o
pulm/o	thym/o
rect/o	thyr/o
rhin/o	trache/o
salping/o	ur/o
splen/o	urethr/o
stern/o	urin/o
stomat/o	uter/o

chest	mind
thymus	lung
thyroid	rectum
trachea	nose
urine, urinary tract, urination	auditory (eustachian) tube, uterine (fallopian) tube
urethra	spleen
urine	sternum
uterus	mouth

ven/o	thromb/o
fibr/o	tox/o, toxic/o
glyc/o	a—
gynec/o	ante—
hydr/o	anti—
lith/o	bio—
ped/o	brady—
py/o	contra—

clot	vein
poison	fiber
without	sugar
before	woman
against, counteracting	water
life	stone
slow	child
against, opposed	pus

dys—	poly—
hyper—	pre—
hypo—	pseudo—
inter—	tachy—
intra—	—centesis
neo—	—genic
pan—	—gram
peri—	—logy

many	pain or difficulty
before	above, excessive
false	low, deficient
fast	between
puncture or aspiration of	within
producing, causing	new
record	all
study of	around

—lysis	—rrhagia
—megaly	—rrhea
—otomy	—scope
—pathy	—scopy
—penia	—stasis
—plegia	
—pnea	
—ptosis	

excessive flow	destruction
profuse flow, discharge	enlargement
examination instrument	incision
examination using a scope	disease
maintaining a constant level	lack, deficiency
	paralysis
	breathing, respiration
	falling, sagging, dropping down